The Complete
GOOD ENERGY
Cookbook for Beginners

1,200 Days of Healthy, Metabolism-Boosting, Weight-Loss Good Energy Recipes Inspired by Dr. Casey Means' Table Tenet (30-Day Meal Plan)

Aisha Wilson

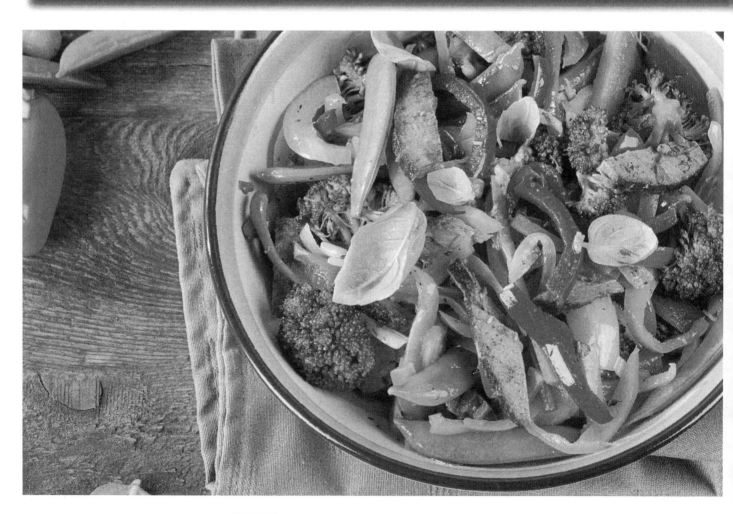

CONTENTS

Chapter 1 Introduction

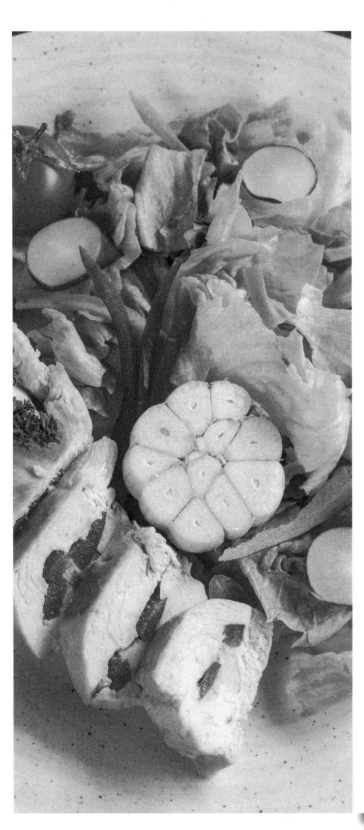

Overview

The Good Energy diet is a transformative approach to nutrition, designed to enhance energy levels and promote overall health through the consumption of whole, nutrient-dense foods. This dietary philosophy was developed based on the teachings of Dr. Casey Means, a prominent figure in nutritional science and holistic health. Dr. Means emphasizes that our dietary choices significantly impact our physical vitality, mental clarity, and emotional well-being, encouraging a shift towards wholesome eating habits.

The concept behind the Good Energy diet is simple yet profound: the food we eat directly affects our body's energy production, mood, and long-term health. By focusing on high-quality ingredients and balanced meals, this diet empowers individuals to reclaim their vitality and foster a healthier relationship with food. As a result, many who adopt the Good Energy diet experience remarkable improvements in their overall well-being, demonstrating the profound connection between nutrition and health.

Origins of the Good Energy Diet

Dr. Casey Means's journey to creating the Good Energy diet began with her passion for understanding the intricate relationship between food and health. She has a background in medicine, and her experiences in clinical practice led her to realize that many health issues are linked to poor dietary choices. Through extensive research and clinical experience, she formulated the principles of the Good Energy diet, which emphasizes the importance of selecting foods that provide sustained energy rather than those that lead to quick spikes and crashes in blood sugar levels.

Dr. Means's insights are rooted in scientific research that highlights how certain foods can optimize the body's performance, enhance mood, and even prevent chronic diseases. The Good Energy diet was introduced through her influential work, particularly in her book "The Table of Good Energy," where she outlines the vision of a diet that goes beyond mere calorie counting to focus on nourishing the body with high-quality, unprocessed foods. This dietary framework not only addresses physical health but also mental and emotional well-being, creating a holistic approach to nutrition that resonates with many individuals

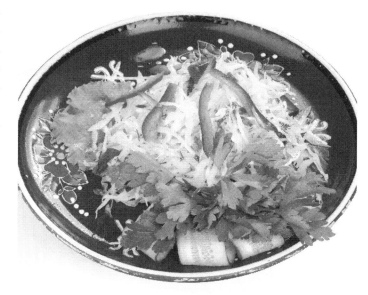

Benefits of the Good Energy Diet

The Good Energy diet offers a multitude of benefits that cater to various aspects of health. Each benefit contributes to a comprehensive improvement in one's quality of life, making this dietary approach an attractive option for those seeking lasting health changes:

1.Increased Energy Levels: By prioritizing whole foods that release energy slowly, this diet prevents the energy crashes often experienced with processed foods high in refined sugars. Individuals following the Good Energy diet frequently report sustained energy throughout the day, enabling them to engage in their daily activities with vigor and enthusiasm. Unlike traditional diets that may leave individuals feeling sluggish, the Good Energy diet helps maintain stable blood sugar levels, promoting a steady energy supply.

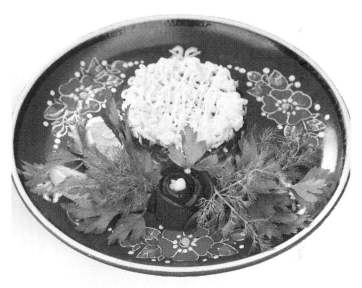

2.Enhanced Mental Clarity and Mood: The diet incorporates nutrient-rich foods such as omega-3 fatty acids, antioxidants, and fiber, which support brain health and cognitive function. Many individuals notice significant improvements in their mood and mental clarity after adopting the Good Energy diet, experiencing reduced anxiety and mood swings. Research has shown that certain nutrients, like omega-3s found in fatty fish, can play a crucial role in improving mood and cognitive function, leading to better emotional health overall.

3.Weight Management Support: The Good Energy diet promotes healthier eating habits through the consumption

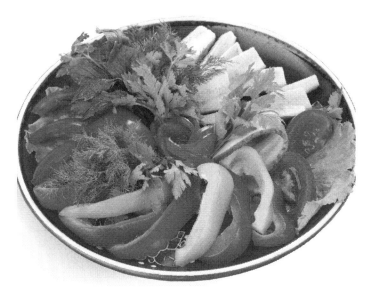

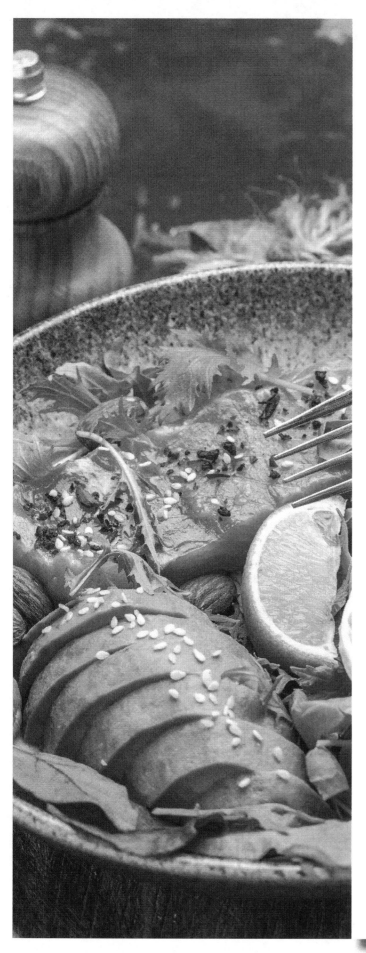

of whole foods that are high in fiber and low in empty calories. Many individuals find it easier to maintain a healthy weight while following this diet, as they feel more satiated and are less likely to indulge in unhealthy snacking. The emphasis on portion control and balanced meals helps prevent overeating, contributing to long-term weight management success.

4.Improved Digestive Health: The inclusion of a variety of fruits, vegetables, and whole grains contributes to better gut health. The high fiber content in these foods aids digestion, reduces bloating, and promotes regular bowel movements. Research indicates that a diet rich in fiber can lead to a healthier gut microbiome, which is crucial for overall digestive health and can even influence mood and immune function.

5.Lowered Risk of Chronic Diseases: Research consistently shows that diets rich in plant-based foods and healthy fats are linked to a decreased incidence of chronic diseases, such as heart disease, diabetes, and certain cancers. The Good Energy diet aligns with these findings by encouraging the consumption of nutrient-dense foods that support overall health and longevity. A growing body of evidence suggests that diets high in fruits, vegetables, and whole grains can significantly reduce the risk of developing chronic health conditions.

6.Sustainable Eating Practices: The Good Energy diet promotes not only personal health but also environmental sustainability. By emphasizing whole, minimally processed foods, individuals are encouraged to make conscious choices about their food sources. This often leads to increased consumption of local and seasonal produce, which can reduce the carbon footprint associated with food transportation. Additionally, supporting local farmers and sustainable agriculture practices can foster a stronger community connection and promote healthier ecosystems.

7.Holistic Wellness: This diet does not only focus on physical health; it also emphasizes emotional and mental well-being. The act of preparing and enjoying wholesome meals can serve as a mindful practice that enhances one's relationship with food. Mindful eating encourages individuals to be present during meals, promoting gratitude for the nourishment they receive and fostering a healthier mindset towards food.

Important Considerations for Following Good Energy Nutrition

While Good Energy nutrition offers numerous advantages, several key considerations should be kept in mind to maximize its benefits:

1.Emphasize Whole Foods: Focus on consuming fresh fruits, vegetables, whole grains, lean proteins, and healthy fats. Avoid processed and refined foods that can detract from the benefits of this diet.

2.Balance Macronutrients: Ensure a proper balance of carbohydrates, proteins, and fats in your meals. Each macronutrient plays a critical role in maintaining energy levels and supporting metabolic functions.

3.Stay Hydrated: Proper hydration is essential for energy management and optimal metabolic function. Aim to drink plenty of water and include hydrating foods like cucumbers, watermelon, and leafy greens in your diet.

4.Listen to Your Body: Pay attention to hunger and satiety cues. Good Energy nutrition encourages intuitive eating, helping individuals develop a better understanding of their nutritional needs and preferences.

5.Meal Planning: To stay on track with dietary goals, consider meal planning and preparation. Having healthy meals and snacks readily available can prevent impulsive choices that may not align with the principles of Good Energy nutrition.

6.Practice Mindful Eating: Engage in mindful eating by savoring each bite and minimizing distractions during meals. This can enhance the enjoyment of food and improve digestion.

7.Consult a Professional: If you have specific health concerns or dietary restrictions, consider consulting with a registered dietitian or healthcare professional to tailor the Good Energy diet to your individual needs.

8.Be Patient and Flexible: Adopting a new dietary approach can take time. Be patient with yourself and

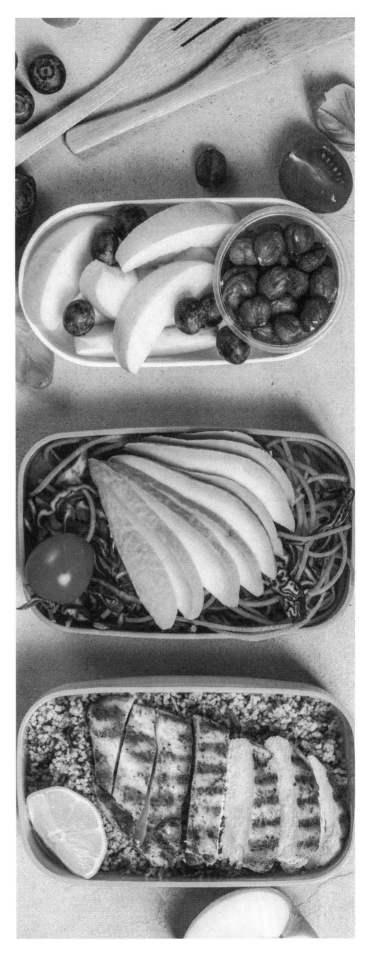

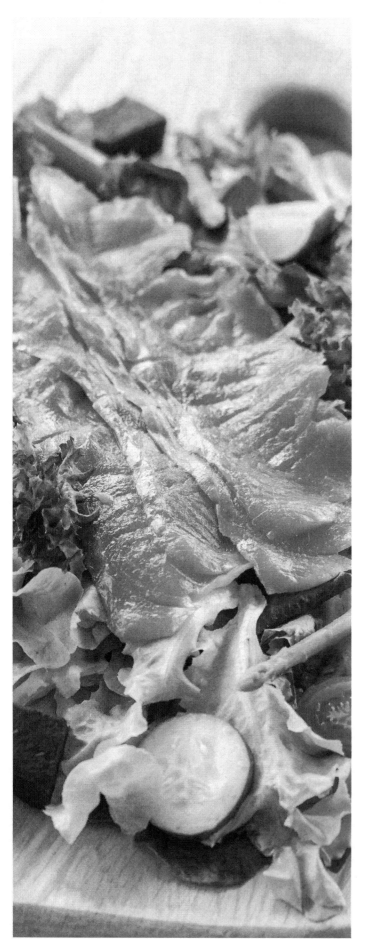

allow for flexibility as you transition into the Good Energy lifestyle.

Scientific Research Supporting Good Energy Nutrition

Numerous scientific studies support the principles of Good Energy nutrition, demonstrating the health benefits of a diet rich in whole, nutrient-dense foods.

1.Impact on Metabolic Health: Research published in the Journal of Nutrition indicates that diets high in whole foods, particularly fruits, vegetables, whole grains, and lean proteins, can significantly improve markers of metabolic health. A study involving participants with prediabetes found that those following a whole food diet experienced improvements in insulin sensitivity and reductions in inflammatory markers compared to those consuming a typical Western diet.

2.Sustained Energy Levels: A study in the American Journal of Clinical Nutrition examined the effects of different carbohydrate sources on energy levels. The findings revealed that complex carbohydrates from whole grains and legumes led to sustained energy levels and improved mood, while simple carbohydrates from sugary foods resulted in energy spikes followed by crashes.

3.Weight Management: A meta-analysis published in Obesity Reviews found that diets rich in whole foods are associated with greater weight loss and weight maintenance compared to diets that include processed foods. Participants in these studies reported feeling fuller and more satisfied when consuming whole foods, reducing the likelihood of overeating.

4.Cognitive Function: Research published in Frontiers in Aging Neuroscience suggests that diets rich in antioxidants and healthy fats, such as the Mediterranean diet, can protect against cognitive decline. Foods high in omega-3 fatty acids, such as fatty fish and walnuts, are particularly beneficial for brain health.

Case Studies Demonstrating the Benefits of Good Energy Nutrition

1.Case Study: Sarah's Transformation: Sarah, a 34-year-old marketing professional, struggled with fatigue and weight gain for years. After being introduced to Good Energy nutrition by her registered dietitian, she shifted her focus to whole foods and began practicing mindful eating. Over six months, Sarah lost 25 pounds, reported improved energy levels, and experienced better focus at work. Her experience underscores the power of nutrient-dense foods in enhancing daily vitality and overall well-being.

2.Case Study: John's Diabetes Reversal: John, a 52-year-old man with type 2 diabetes, faced challenges managing his blood sugar levels with conventional treatments. Upon adopting the Good Energy diet, which included an increased intake of vegetables, whole grains, and healthy fats, he saw remarkable improvements. His HbA1c levels dropped from 8.2% to 6.5% within a year, and he was able to reduce his reliance on medication. John's case highlights how a whole-food, nutrient-focused diet can have profound effects on metabolic health.

Case Study: Lisa's Mental Clarity: Lisa, a 28-year-old graduate student, often struggled with concentration and mental fog. After integrating Good Energy principles into her diet, she noted significant changes in her cognitive function. By focusing on foods rich in antioxidants and omega-3 fatty acids, she improved her mental clarity and focus, leading to better academic performance. Her story illustrates how proper nutrition can enhance cognitive abilities and emotional well-being.

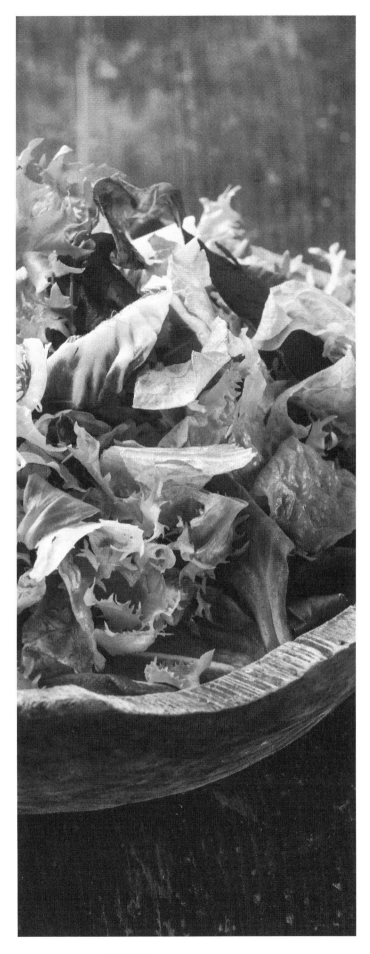

Chapter 2 30 Day Meal Plan

DAY	BREAKFAST	LUNCH	DINNER
1	Quinoa Breakfast Bowl with Berries 15	Quinoa Salad with Chickpeas and Avocado 21	Lemon Herb Grilled Chicken with Quinoa 27
2	Savory Sweet Potato and Spinach Hash 15	Stuffed Bell Peppers with Quinoa and Black Beans 21	Vegetable Stir-Fry with Brown Rice 27
3	Overnight Oats with Almond Butter and Banana 16	Lentil Soup with Spinach and Carrots 22	Baked Salmon with Asparagus 27
4	Chickpea Flour Pancakes with Spinach and Feta 16	Zucchini Noodles with Pesto and Cherry Tomatoes 22	Baked Cod with Lemon and Garlic 31
5	Greek Yogurt Parfait with Nuts and Seeds 16	Baked Sweet Potato with Black Bean Salsa 22	Stuffed Bell Peppers with Quinoa and Turkey 28
6	Avocado Toast with Cherry Tomatoes and Basil 16	Chickpea Salad with Cucumber and Feta 22	Zucchini Noodles with Turkey Meatballs 28
7	Zucchini and Carrot Fritters 17	Mushroom and Spinach Quinoa Bowl 23	Chickpea Curry with Brown Rice 28
8	Oven-Baked Egg Muffins with Vegetables 17	Cauliflower Rice Stir-Fry 23	Moroccan Lentil Stew 31
9	Fruit and Nut Smoothie Bowl 17	Mediterranean Tuna Salad 23	Spaghetti Squash with Roasted Vegetables 29
10	Baked Apples with Cinnamon and Walnuts 18	Sweet Potato and Kale Hash 24	Cilantro Lime Shrimp with Cauliflower Rice 29
11	Millet Porridge with Nuts and Dried Fruit 18	Asian-Inspired Quinoa Bowl 24	Sweet Potato and Black Bean Tacos 29
12	Coconut Chia Seed Pudding 18	Egg and Avocado Wrap 24	Eggplant and Chickpea Stew 30
13	Roasted Vegetable and Hummus Toast 18	Roasted Vegetable Quinoa Salad 25	Grilled Portobello Mushrooms with Pesto 30
14	Vegetable Omelette with Herbs 19	Cabbage and Carrot Slaw with Sesame Dressing 25	Oven-Baked Chicken Fajitas 30
15	Raspberry Almond Overnight Oats 19	Spaghetti Squash with Marinara Sauce 25	Cauliflower and Chickpea Salad 31

DAY	BREAKFAST	LUNCH	DINNER
16	Quinoa Breakfast Bowl with Berries 15	Quinoa Salad with Chickpeas and Avocado 21	Lemon Herb Grilled Chicken with Quinoa 27
17	Savory Sweet Potato and Spinach Hash 15	Stuffed Bell Peppers with Quinoa and Black Beans 21	Vegetable Stir-Fry with Brown Rice 27
18	Overnight Oats with Almond Butter and Banana 16	Lentil Soup with Spinach and Carrots 22	Baked Salmon with Asparagus 27
19	Chickpea Flour Pancakes with Spinach and Feta 16	Zucchini Noodles with Pesto and Cherry Tomatoes 22	Baked Cod with Lemon and Garlic 31
20	Greek Yogurt Parfait with Nuts and Seeds 16	Baked Sweet Potato with Black Bean Salsa 22	Stuffed Bell Peppers with Quinoa and Turkey 28
21	Avocado Toast with Cherry Tomatoes and Basil 16	Chickpea Salad with Cucumber and Feta 22	Zucchini Noodles with Turkey Meatballs 28
22	Zucchini and Carrot Fritters 17	Mushroom and Spinach Quinoa Bowl 23	Chickpea Curry with Brown Rice 28
23	Oven-Baked Egg Muffins with Vegetables 17	Cauliflower Rice Stir-Fry 23	Moroccan Lentil Stew 31
24	Fruit and Nut Smoothie Bowl 17	Mediterranean Tuna Salad 23	Spaghetti Squash with Roasted Vegetables 29
25	Baked Apples with Cinnamon and Walnuts 18	Sweet Potato and Kale Hash 24	Cilantro Lime Shrimp with Cauliflower Rice 29
26	Millet Porridge with Nuts and Dried Fruit 18	Asian-Inspired Quinoa Bowl 24	Sweet Potato and Black Bean Tacos 29
27	Coconut Chia Seed Pudding 18	Egg and Avocado Wrap 24	Eggplant and Chickpea Stew 30
28	Roasted Vegetable and Hummus Toast 18	Roasted Vegetable Quinoa Salad 25	Grilled Portobello Mushrooms with Pesto 30
29	Vegetable Omelette with Herbs 19	Cabbage and Carrot Slaw with Sesame Dressing 25	Oven-Baked Chicken Fajitas 30
30	Raspberry Almond Overnight Oats 19	Spaghetti Squash with Marinara Sauce 25	Cauliflower and Chickpea Salad 31

Chapter 3 Measurement Conversions

BASIC KITCHEN CONVERSIONS & EQUIVALENTS

DRY MEASUREMENTS CONVERSION CHART
3 TEASPOONS = 1 TABLESPOON = 1/16 CUP
6 TEASPOONS = 2 TABLESPOONS = 1/8 CUP
12 TEASPOONS = 4 TABLESPOONS = 1/4 CUP
24 TEASPOONS = 8 TABLESPOONS = 1/2 CUP
36 TEASPOONS = 12 TABLESPOONS = 3/4 CUP
48 TEASPOONS = 16 TABLESPOONS = 1 CUP

METRIC TO US COOKING CONVERSIONS

BAKING PAN CONVERSIONS
9-INCH ROUND CAKE PAN = 12 CUPS
10-INCH TUBE PAN = 16 CUPS
11-INCH BUNDT PAN = 12 CUPS
9-INCH SPRINGFORM PAN = 10 CUPS
9 X 5 INCH LOAF PAN = 8 CUPS
9-INCH SQUARE PAN = 8 CUPS

BUTTER
1 CUP BUTTER = 2 STICKS = 8 OUNCES = 230 GRAMS = 8 TABLESPOONS

WEIGHT
1 GRAM = .035 OUNCES
100 GRAMS = 3.5 OUNCES
500 GRAMS = 1.1 POUNDS
1 KILOGRAM = 35 OUNCES

BAKING IN GRAMS

1 CUP FLOUR = 140 GRAMS	
1 CUP SUGAR = 150 GRAMS	
1 CUP POWDERED SUGAR = 160 GRAMS	
1 CUP HEAVY CREAM = 235 GRAMS	

US TO METRIC COOKING CONVERSIONS

1/5 TSP = 1 ML
1 TSP = 5 ML
1 TBSP = 15 ML
1 FL OUNCE = 30 ML
1 CUP = 237 ML
1 PINT (2 CUPS) = 473 ML
1 QUART (4 CUPS) = .95 LITER
1 GALLON (16 CUPS) = 3.8 LITERS
1 OZ = 28 GRAMS
1 POUND = 454 GRAMS

VOLUME

1 MILLILITER = 1/5 TEASPOON
5 ML = 1 TEASPOON
15 ML = 1 TABLESPOON
240 ML = 1 CUP OR 8 FLUID OUNCES
1 LITER = 34 FL. OUNCES

BAKING PAN CONVERSIONS

1 CUP ALL-PURPOSE FLOUR = 4.5 OZ
1 CUP ROLLED OATS = 3 OZ 1 LARGE EGG = 1.7 OZ
1 CUP BUTTER = 8 OZ 1 CUP MILK = 8 OZ
1 CUP HEAVY CREAM = 8.4 OZ
1 CUP GRANULATED SUGAR = 7.1 OZ
1 CUP PACKED BROWN SUGAR = 7.75 OZ
1 CUP VEGETABLE OIL = 7.7 OZ
1 CUP UNSIFTED POWDERED SUGAR = 4.4 OZ

LIQUID MEASUREMENTS CONVERSION CHART

8 FLUID OUNCES = 1 CUP = 1/2 PINT = 1/4 QUART
16 FLUID OUNCES = 2 CUPS = 1 PINT = 1/2 QUART
32 FLUID OUNCES = 4 CUPS = 2 PINTS = 1 QUART = 1/4 GALLON
128 FLUID OUNCES = 16 CUPS = 8 PINTS = 4 QUARTS = 1 GALLON

OVEN TEMPERATURES

120 °C = 250 °F
160 °C = 320 °F
180° C = 350 °F
205 °C = 400 °F
220 °C = 425 °F

Chapter 4 Breakfast Recipes

Chapter 4 Breakfast Recipes

Quinoa Breakfast Bowl with Berries

Benefits: This quinoa breakfast bowl is rich in antioxidants from the berries and packed with protein from the quinoa and chia seeds, making it a perfect start to your day.

Servings: 2
Preparation Time: 10 minutes
Cooking Time: 15 minutes

Ingredients:

- 1 cup quinoa
- 2 cups almond milk (unsweetened)
- 1 cup mixed berries (blueberries, strawberries, raspberries)
- 1 tablespoon chia seeds
- 1 tablespoon honey or maple syrup (optional)
- 1 teaspoon vanilla extract
- 1 tablespoon chopped almonds

Instructions:

1. Rinse the quinoa under cold water to remove its natural coating, which can be bitter.
2. In a saucepan, combine the rinsed quinoa and almond milk. Bring to a boil, then reduce heat to low, cover, and simmer for 15 minutes until the quinoa is fluffy and liquid is absorbed.
3. Remove from heat and stir in the chia seeds, vanilla extract, and honey or maple syrup if using.
4. Divide the quinoa into bowls and top with mixed berries and chopped almonds. Serve warm.

Nutritional Information (per serving):

- Calories: 290; Fat: 9g; Protein: 9g; Carbs: 45g

Savory Sweet Potato and Spinach Hash

Benefits: This colorful hash is a great source of vitamins A and C from sweet potatoes and spinach, providing energy and supporting immune health.

Servings: 2
Preparation Time: 10 minutes
Cooking Time: 20 minutes

Ingredients:

- 2 medium sweet potatoes, diced
- 2 cups fresh spinach
- 1 small onion, chopped
- 2 cloves garlic, minced
- 1 tablespoon olive oil
- Salt and pepper to taste
- 2 eggs (optional)

Instructions:

1. Heat olive oil in a large skillet over medium heat. Add the diced sweet potatoes and cook for about 10 minutes, stirring occasionally until they start to soften.
2. Add the chopped onion and minced garlic, cooking for an additional 5 minutes until the onion is translucent.
3. Stir in the fresh spinach and cook until wilted. Season with salt and pepper.
4. If using, fry or poach eggs to serve on top of the hash.

Nutritional Information (per serving without eggs):

- Calories: 220; Fat: 7g; Protein: 5g; Carbs: 37g

Overnight Oats with Almond Butter and Banana

Benefits: Overnight oats are an excellent source of fiber and healthy fats, providing sustained energy throughout the morning.

Servings: 2
Preparation Time: 5 minutes
Cooking Time: 0 minutes (overnight soak)

Ingredients:

- 1 cup rolled oats
- 2 cups almond milk (unsweetened)
- 2 tablespoons almond butter
- 1 banana, sliced
- 1 tablespoon chia seeds
- 1 teaspoon cinnamon

Instructions:

1. In a bowl or jar, combine rolled oats, almond milk, chia seeds, and cinnamon. Mix well.
2. Cover and refrigerate overnight.
3. In the morning, stir the oats, adding more almond milk if needed for desired consistency. Top with almond butter and banana slices before serving.

Nutritional Information (per serving):

- Calories: 350; Fat: 14g; Protein: 10g; Carbs: 54g

Chickpea Flour Pancakes with Spinach and Feta

Benefits: These protein-packed pancakes are a fantastic alternative to traditional pancakes, providing complex carbohydrates and essential nutrients.

Servings: 2
Preparation Time: 10 minutes
Cooking Time: 10 minutes

Ingredients:

- 1 cup chickpea flour
- 1 cup water
- 1 cup fresh spinach, chopped
- 1/4 cup feta cheese, crumbled
- 1 tablespoon olive oil
- Salt and pepper to taste

Instructions:

1. In a bowl, mix chickpea flour with water to create a batter. Add salt and pepper to taste.
2. Stir in chopped spinach and feta cheese.

3. Heat olive oil in a skillet over medium heat. Pour batter to form pancakes, cooking for 3-4 minutes on each side until golden.
4. Serve warm with a side salad or yogurt.

Nutritional Information (per serving):

- Calories: 320; Fat: 15g; Protein: 20g; Carbs: 30g

Greek Yogurt Parfait with Nuts and Seeds

Benefits: This parfait offers a balanced meal with probiotics from the yogurt, healthy fats from nuts, and vitamins from fruit.

Servings: 2
Preparation Time: 5 minutes
Cooking Time: 0 minutes

Ingredients:

- 2 cups plain Greek yogurt (unsweetened)
- 1/2 cup mixed nuts (almonds, walnuts, pecans)
- 1/4 cup sunflower seeds
- 1 cup fresh fruit (berries, peaches, or apples)
- 1 tablespoon honey or maple syrup (optional)

Instructions:

1. In two glasses or bowls, layer Greek yogurt, fresh fruit, mixed nuts, and sunflower seeds.
2. Drizzle with honey or maple syrup if desired.
3. Repeat the layers and serve immediately.

Nutritional Information (per serving):

- Calories: 400; Fat: 20g; Protein: 30g; Carbs: 35g

Avocado Toast with Cherry Tomatoes and Basil

Benefits: This vibrant toast is high in healthy fats and fiber, making it filling and nutrient-dense for a satisfying breakfast.

Servings: 2
Preparation Time: 10 minutes
Cooking Time: 0 minutes

Ingredients:

- 2 slices whole-grain bread
- 1 ripe avocado
- 1 cup cherry tomatoes, halved
- Fresh basil leaves
- Salt and pepper to taste
- 1 tablespoon balsamic vinegar (optional)

Instructions:

1. Toast the whole-grain bread slices until golden.
2. In a bowl, mash the avocado and season with salt and pepper.
3. Spread the mashed avocado on each slice of toast.
4. Top with halved cherry tomatoes and fresh basil leaves. Drizzle with balsamic vinegar if using.

Nutritional Information (per serving):

- Calories: 310; Fat: 20g; Protein: 8g; Carbs: 30g

Zucchini and Carrot Fritters

Benefits: These fritters are an excellent way to sneak in vegetables while enjoying a delicious breakfast packed with fiber and protein.

Servings: 2
Preparation Time: 15 minutes
Cooking Time: 15 minutes

Ingredients:

- 1 medium zucchini, grated
- 1 medium carrot, grated
- 2 eggs
- 1/4 cup almond flour
- 1 teaspoon garlic powder
- Salt and pepper to taste
- Olive oil for frying

Instructions:

1. In a bowl, mix grated zucchini, grated carrot, eggs, almond flour, garlic powder, salt, and pepper.
2. Heat olive oil in a skillet over medium heat. Drop spoonfuls of the mixture into the skillet, flattening them slightly.
3. Cook for 3-4 minutes on each side until golden brown.
4. Serve warm with a yogurt dip or fresh salsa.

Nutritional Information (per serving):

- Calories: 280; Fat: 18g; Protein: 12g; Carbs: 20g

Oven-Baked Egg Muffins with Vegetables

Benefits: These egg muffins are a convenient, portable breakfast option that's high in protein and low in carbs, making them great for meal prep.

Servings: 4
Preparation Time: 10 minutes

Cooking Time: 20 minutes

Ingredients:

- 8 large eggs
- 1/2 cup bell peppers, diced
- 1/2 cup spinach, chopped
- 1/4 cup onion, diced
- 1/4 cup feta cheese (optional)

Salt and pepper to taste

Instructions:

1. Preheat the oven to 350°F (175°C).
2. In a bowl, whisk the eggs and season with salt and pepper.
3. Stir in the diced bell peppers, chopped spinach, onion, and feta cheese if using.
4. Pour the mixture into a greased muffin tin, filling each cup about 3/4 full.
5. Bake for 15-20 minutes, or until the eggs are set. Let cool slightly before removing.

Nutritional Information (per muffin, makes 12):

- Calories: 80; Fat: 5g; Protein: 7g; Carbs: 2g

Fruit and Nut Smoothie Bowl

Benefits: This smoothie bowl is refreshing and energizing, loaded with vitamins, minerals, and healthy fats to keep you full and satisfied.

Servings: 2
Preparation Time: 10 minutes
Cooking Time: 0 minutes

Ingredients:

- 1 banana
- 1 cup spinach
- 1/2 cup unsweetened almond milk
- 1/2 cup mixed berries
- 2 tablespoons almond butter
- 1 tablespoon chia seeds
- Toppings: sliced banana, berries, and chopped nuts

Instructions:

1. In a blender, combine banana, spinach, almond milk, mixed berries, almond butter, and chia seeds. Blend until smooth.
2. Pour the smoothie into bowls and top with additional banana slices, berries, and chopped nuts.

Nutritional Information (per serving):

- Calories: 320; Fat: 15g; Protein: 10g; Carbs: 45g

Baked Apples with Cinnamon and Walnuts

Benefits: These baked apples are a warm, comforting breakfast that's naturally sweetened and high in fiber, perfect for a cozy morning.

Servings: 2
Preparation Time: 10 minutes
Cooking Time: 30 minutes

Ingredients:

- 2 large apples, cored
- 1/4 cup walnuts, chopped
- 1 teaspoon cinnamon
- 1 tablespoon honey or maple syrup (optional)
- 1 tablespoon raisins (optional)

Instructions:

1. Preheat the oven to 350°F (175°C).
2. In a bowl, mix chopped walnuts, cinnamon, honey or maple syrup, and raisins if using.
3. Stuff the mixture into the cored apples.
4. Place the apples in a baking dish and add a splash of water to the bottom. Bake for 30 minutes until tender.

Nutritional Information (per serving):

- Calories: 250; Fat: 10g; Protein: 3g; Carbs: 40g

Millet Porridge with Nuts and Dried Fruit

Benefits: Millet is a gluten-free grain that's rich in fiber and minerals, making this porridge a wholesome breakfast option.

Servings: 2
Preparation Time: 5 minutes
Cooking Time: 20 minutes

Ingredients:

- 1 cup millet
- 2 cups water
- 1/4 cup mixed nuts, chopped
- 1/4 cup dried fruit (raisins, cranberries, or apricots)
- 1 tablespoon honey or maple syrup (optional)
- 1 teaspoon vanilla extract

Instructions:

1. Rinse the millet under cold water.
2. In a saucepan, combine millet and water. Bring to a boil, then reduce heat, cover, and simmer for 15-20 minutes until the millet is tender and water is absorbed.

3. Stir in nuts, dried fruit, honey or maple syrup, and vanilla extract. Serve warm.

Nutritional Information (per serving):

- Calories: 350; Fat: 10g; Protein: 10g; Carbs: 60g

Coconut Chia Seed Pudding

Benefits: This chia seed pudding is packed with omega-3 fatty acids and fiber, making it a nutritious and satisfying breakfast option.

Servings: 2
Preparation Time: 5 minutes
Cooking Time: 0 minutes (overnight soak)

Ingredients:

- 1/2 cup chia seeds
- 2 cups coconut milk (unsweetened)
- 1 teaspoon vanilla extract
- 1 tablespoon maple syrup or honey (optional)
- Fresh fruit for topping (mango, kiwi, berries)

Instructions:

1. In a bowl or jar, mix chia seeds, coconut milk, vanilla extract, and sweetener if using.
2. Stir well to prevent clumping, then cover and refrigerate overnight.
3. In the morning, stir the pudding again and top with fresh fruit before serving.

Nutritional Information (per serving):

- Calories: 320; Fat: 25g; Protein: 5g; Carbs: 30g

Roasted Vegetable and Hummus Toast

Benefits: This hearty toast is packed with fiber and plant-based protein, making it a satisfying and energizing breakfast.

Servings: 2
Preparation Time: 15 minutes
Cooking Time: 20 minutes

Ingredients:

- 1 cup mixed vegetables (bell peppers, zucchini, eggplant), diced
- 2 slices whole-grain bread
- 1/2 cup hummus (store-bought or homemade)
- 1 tablespoon olive oil
- Salt and pepper to taste

Instructions:

1. Preheat the oven to 400°F (200°C).

2. Toss the mixed vegetables with olive oil, salt, and pepper. Spread them on a baking sheet and roast for 20 minutes until tender.
3. Toast the whole-grain bread.
4. Spread hummus on each slice of toast and top with roasted vegetables.

Nutritional Information (per serving):
- Calories: 330; Fat: 10g; Protein: 12g; Carbs: 45g

Vegetable Omelette with Herbs

Benefits: This omelette is a protein powerhouse, providing essential nutrients while keeping carbs low for sustained energy.

Servings: 2
Preparation Time: 10 minutes
Cooking Time: 10 minutes

Ingredients:
- 4 large eggs
- 1/2 cup bell peppers, diced
- 1/2 cup mushrooms, sliced
- 1/4 cup onion, diced
- 1 tablespoon fresh herbs (parsley, chives, or basil)
- Salt and pepper to taste
- Olive oil for cooking

Instructions:

1. In a bowl, whisk the eggs and season with salt and pepper.
2. Heat olive oil in a skillet over medium heat. Add diced bell peppers, mushrooms, and onion, cooking until softened.
3. Pour the whisked eggs over the vegetables, tilting the pan to distribute evenly. Cook until the edges set, then fold in half.
4. Cook for an additional 1-2 minutes until fully set. Serve topped with fresh herbs.

Nutritional Information (per serving):
- Calories: 220; Fat: 15g; Protein: 18g; Carbs: 4g

Raspberry Almond Overnight Oats

Benefits: This overnight oats recipe is rich in fiber and healthy fats, providing a deliciously satisfying breakfast that keeps you full longer.

Servings: 2
Preparation Time: 5 minutes
Cooking Time: 0 minutes (overnight soak)

Ingredients:
- 1 cup rolled oats
- 2 cups almond milk (unsweetened)
- 1 cup raspberries (fresh or frozen)
- 2 tablespoons almond butter
- 1 tablespoon flax seeds
- 1 tablespoon maple syrup (optional)

Instructions:

1. In a bowl or jar, combine rolled oats, almond milk, flax seeds, and maple syrup if using. Mix well.
2. Stir in half of the raspberries. Cover and refrigerate overnight.
3. In the morning, stir the oats and top with almond butter and remaining raspberries.

Nutritional Information (per serving):
- Calories: 350; Fat: 15g; Protein: 10g; Carbs: 50g

Chapter 5 Lunch Recipes

Chapter 5 Lunch Recipes

Quinoa Salad with Chickpeas and Avocado

Benefits: This salad is a complete meal packed with protein, fiber, and healthy fats, providing sustained energy and keeping you full longer.

Servings: 4
Preparation Time: 15 minutes
Cooking Time: 15 minutes

Ingredients:

- 1 cup quinoa
- 2 cups water
- 1 can (15 oz) chickpeas, drained and rinsed
- 1 ripe avocado, diced
- 1 cup cherry tomatoes, halved
- 1/4 cup red onion, diced
- 1/4 cup fresh parsley, chopped
- 3 tablespoons olive oil
- Juice of 1 lemon
- Salt and pepper to taste

Instructions:

1. Rinse the quinoa under cold water. In a saucepan, combine quinoa and water; bring to a boil.
2. Reduce heat, cover, and simmer for 15 minutes or until quinoa is fluffy and water is absorbed.
3. In a large bowl, combine the cooked quinoa, chickpeas, avocado, cherry tomatoes, red onion, and parsley.
4. In a small bowl, whisk together olive oil, lemon juice, salt, and pepper. Pour over the salad and toss gently.
5. Serve chilled or at room temperature.

Nutritional Information (per serving):

- Calories: 380; Fat: 16g; Protein: 12g; Carbs: 50g

Stuffed Bell Peppers with Quinoa and Black Beans

Benefits: These stuffed peppers are colorful and satisfying, providing a balance of protein and complex carbohydrates, making them a perfect midday meal.

Servings: 4
Preparation Time: 20 minutes
Cooking Time: 30 minutes

Ingredients:

- 4 bell peppers (any color)
- 1 cup cooked quinoa
- 1 can (15 oz) black beans, drained and rinsed
- 1 cup corn (fresh or frozen)
- 1 teaspoon cumin
- 1 teaspoon paprika
- 1/2 teaspoon salt
- 1/4 teaspoon black pepper
- 1 cup salsa

Instructions:

1. Preheat the oven to 375°F (190°C).
2. Cut the tops off the bell peppers and remove seeds.
3. In a bowl, mix quinoa, black beans, corn, cumin, paprika, salt, and pepper.
4. Stuff each pepper with the quinoa mixture and place in a baking dish.
5. Pour salsa over the peppers and cover with foil. Bake for 25 minutes, then uncover and bake for an additional 5 minutes.
6. Serve warm.

Nutritional Information (per serving):

- Calories: 320; Fat: 4g; Protein: 14g; Carbs: 60g

Lentil Soup with Spinach and Carrots

Benefits: This hearty soup is rich in protein and fiber, making it a comforting and nutritious option that warms you from the inside out.

Servings: 4
Preparation Time: 10 minutes
Cooking Time: 30 minutes

Ingredients:

- 1 cup dried lentils, rinsed
- 1 onion, chopped
- 2 carrots, diced
- 2 cups fresh spinach
- 3 cloves garlic, minced
- 1 teaspoon thyme
- 1 teaspoon cumin
- 6 cups vegetable broth
- Salt and pepper to taste

Instructions:

1. In a large pot, sauté onions and garlic until fragrant.
2. Add carrots and cook for another 5 minutes.
3. Stir in lentils, thyme, cumin, vegetable broth, salt, and pepper.
4. Bring to a boil, then reduce heat and simmer for 25 minutes until lentils are tender.
5. Stir in fresh spinach and cook for an additional 5 minutes. Serve hot.

Nutritional Information (per serving):

- Calories: 210; Fat: 1g; Protein: 14g; Carbs: 36g

Zucchini Noodles with Pesto and Cherry Tomatoes

Benefits: This dish is a low-carb alternative to traditional pasta, packed with vitamins and healthy fats, making it refreshing and satisfying.

Servings: 2
Preparation Time: 10 minutes
Cooking Time: 5 minutes

Ingredients:

- 2 medium zucchinis, spiralized
- 1 cup cherry tomatoes, halved
- 1/4 cup basil pesto (homemade or store-bought without additives)
- 1 tablespoon olive oil
- Salt and pepper to taste
- Fresh basil leaves for garnish

Instructions:

1. Heat olive oil in a skillet over medium heat. Add spiralized zucchini and sauté for 2-3 minutes until slightly tender.
2. Stir in cherry tomatoes, salt, and pepper, cooking for another 2 minutes.
3. Remove from heat and toss with pesto.
4. Serve garnished with fresh basil leaves.

Nutritional Information (per serving):

- Calories: 220; Fat: 16g; Protein: 4g; Carbs: 20g

Baked Sweet Potato with Black Bean Salsa

Benefits: Baked sweet potatoes are an excellent source of complex carbohydrates and fiber, while the black bean salsa adds protein and flavor, making it a balanced meal.

Servings: 4
Preparation Time: 10 minutes
Cooking Time: 40 minutes

Ingredients:

- 4 medium sweet potatoes
- 1 can (15 oz) black beans, drained and rinsed
- 1 cup corn (fresh or frozen)
- 1/2 cup diced tomatoes
- 1/4 cup cilantro, chopped
- Juice of 1 lime
- Salt and pepper to taste

Instructions:

1. Preheat the oven to 400°F (200°C).
2. Pierce sweet potatoes with a fork and bake for 40 minutes or until tender.
3. In a bowl, mix black beans, corn, diced tomatoes, cilantro, lime juice, salt, and pepper.
4. Once the sweet potatoes are cooked, slice them open and top with the black bean salsa. Serve warm.

Nutritional Information (per serving):

- Calories: 360; Fat: 2g; Protein: 10g; Carbs: 75g

Chickpea Salad with Cucumber and Feta

Benefits: This refreshing salad is rich in protein and healthy fats, making it a perfect light lunch that is both satisfying and nutritious.

Servings: 4
Preparation Time: 15 minutes
Cooking Time: 0 minutes

Ingredients:

- 1 can (15 oz) chickpeas, drained and rinsed
- 1 cucumber, diced
- 1 cup cherry tomatoes, halved
- 1/2 red onion, diced
- 1/4 cup feta cheese, crumbled
- 3 tablespoons olive oil
- Juice of 1 lemon
- Salt and pepper to taste

Instructions:

1. In a large bowl, combine chickpeas, cucumber, cherry tomatoes, red onion, and feta cheese.
2. In a separate bowl, whisk together olive oil, lemon juice, salt, and pepper.
3. Pour the dressing over the salad and toss to combine. Serve immediately or chill in the refrigerator before serving.

Nutritional Information (per serving):

- Calories: 300; Fat: 16g; Protein: 12g; Carbs: 30g

Mushroom and Spinach Quinoa Bowl

Benefits: This bowl is a nutrient-dense meal, offering a great source of plant-based protein, fiber, and essential vitamins from the vegetables.

Servings: 4
Preparation Time: 10 minutes
Cooking Time: 20 minutes

Ingredients:

- 1 cup quinoa
- 2 cups vegetable broth
- 2 cups mushrooms, sliced
- 2 cups spinach
- 2 tablespoons olive oil
- 2 cloves garlic, minced
- Salt and pepper to taste

Instructions:

1. Rinse quinoa under cold water. In a saucepan, combine quinoa and vegetable broth; bring to a boil.
2. Reduce heat, cover, and simmer for 15 minutes until quinoa is fluffy.
3. In a skillet, heat olive oil over medium heat. Add mushrooms and garlic; sauté until mushrooms are tender.
4. Stir in spinach, salt, and pepper, cooking until spinach wilts.
5. Serve the mushroom and spinach mixture over the quinoa.

Nutritional Information (per serving):

- Calories: 280; Fat: 10g; Protein: 10g; Carbs: 40g

Cauliflower Rice Stir-Fry

Benefits: This low-carb stir-fry is a quick and easy meal packed with vegetables, offering a colorful and nutritious option for lunch.

Servings: 4
Preparation Time: 10 minutes
Cooking Time: 15 minutes

Ingredients:

- 1 head cauliflower, grated (or pre-packaged cauliflower rice)
- 1 cup mixed vegetables (carrots, peas, bell peppers)
- 2 cloves garlic, minced
- 3 tablespoons soy sauce (or tamari for gluten-free)
- 1 tablespoon sesame oil
- Green onions for garnish

Instructions:

1. Heat sesame oil in a large skillet over medium heat. Add garlic and mixed vegetables, sautéing for about 5 minutes.
2. Stir in cauliflower rice and soy sauce, cooking for another 5-7 minutes until tender.
3. Garnish with green onions before serving.

Nutritional Information (per serving):

- Calories: 220; Fat: 7g; Protein: 8g; Carbs: 35g

Mediterranean Tuna Salad

Benefits: This protein-packed tuna salad is perfect for a quick lunch, offering heart-healthy fats and a burst of Mediterranean flavors.

Servings: 4
Preparation Time: 10 minutes
Cooking Time: 0 minutes

Ingredients:

- 2 cans (5 oz each) tuna in water, drained
- 1/2 cup cherry tomatoes, halved
- 1/2 cup cucumber, diced
- 1/4 cup red onion, diced
- 1/4 cup olives, sliced

- 2 tablespoons olive oil
- Juice of 1 lemon
- Salt and pepper to taste

Instructions:

1. In a bowl, combine tuna, cherry tomatoes, cucumber, red onion, and olives.
2. In a small bowl, whisk together olive oil, lemon juice, salt, and pepper.
3. Pour the dressing over the tuna mixture and toss gently to combine. Serve on a bed of greens or whole-grain bread.

Nutritional Information (per serving):

- Calories: 250; Fat: 12g; Protein: 30g; Carbs: 8g

Sweet Potato and Kale Hash

Benefits: This hearty hash is a great way to enjoy seasonal vegetables, providing complex carbohydrates and fiber to keep you satisfied.

Servings: 4
Preparation Time: 10 minutes
Cooking Time: 20 minutes

Ingredients:

- 2 medium sweet potatoes, diced
- 2 cups kale, chopped
- 1 onion, diced
- 2 tablespoons olive oil
- 1 teaspoon smoked paprika
- Salt and pepper to taste

Instructions:

1. Heat olive oil in a large skillet over medium heat. Add onion and sweet potatoes; cook for 10 minutes until potatoes are tender.
2. Stir in kale, smoked paprika, salt, and pepper. Cook for an additional 5-7 minutes until kale is wilted. Serve warm.

Nutritional Information (per serving):

- Calories: 280; Fat: 10g; Protein: 4g; Carbs: 44g

Asian-Inspired Quinoa Bowl

Benefits: This bowl is vibrant and packed with nutrients, providing a perfect blend of flavors and textures while supporting your energy levels.

Servings: 4
Preparation Time: 15 minutes
Cooking Time: 15 minutes

Ingredients:

- 1 cup quinoa
- 2 cups vegetable broth
- 1 cup snap peas, trimmed
- 1 cup carrots, julienned
- 1/4 cup soy sauce (or tamari)
- 2 tablespoons sesame oil
- Sesame seeds for garnish

Instructions:

1. Rinse quinoa under cold water. In a saucepan, combine quinoa and vegetable broth; bring to a boil.
2. Reduce heat, cover, and simmer for 15 minutes until quinoa is fluffy.
3. In a skillet, heat sesame oil over medium heat. Add snap peas and carrots; sauté for 5 minutes.
4. Combine quinoa with the vegetables and add soy sauce. Serve warm, garnished with sesame seeds.

Nutritional Information (per serving):

- Calories: 300; Fat: 12g; Protein: 10g; Carbs: 40g

Egg and Avocado Wrap

Benefits: This wrap is a protein-rich meal that combines healthy fats and fiber, perfect for a quick and filling lunch option.

Servings: 2
Preparation Time: 5 minutes
Cooking Time: 5 minutes

Ingredients:

- 4 large eggs
- 2 whole grain tortillas
- 1 ripe avocado, sliced
- 1 cup spinach
- Salt and pepper to taste

Instructions:

1. In a skillet, scramble the eggs until cooked through; season with salt and pepper.
2. Lay the whole grain tortillas flat and fill each with scrambled eggs, avocado slices, and spinach.
3. Roll up the tortillas and serve warm.

Nutritional Information (per serving):

- Calories: 350; Fat: 20g; Protein: 15g; Carbs: 30g

Roasted Vegetable Quinoa Salad

Servings: 4
Preparation Time: 15 minutes
Cooking Time: 25 minutes

Ingredients:

- 1 cup quinoa
- 2 cups vegetable broth
- 1 zucchini, diced
- 1 bell pepper, diced
- 1 red onion, diced
- 2 tablespoons olive oil
- Salt and pepper to taste
- 1/4 cup balsamic vinegar

Instructions:

1. Preheat the oven to 400°F (200°C).
2. Toss zucchini, bell pepper, and red onion with olive oil, salt, and pepper. Spread on a baking sheet and roast for 25 minutes.
3. Meanwhile, rinse quinoa and cook in vegetable broth according to package instructions.
4. In a large bowl, combine roasted vegetables and cooked quinoa. Drizzle with balsamic vinegar and toss gently. Serve warm or cold.

Nutritional Information (per serving):

- Calories: 320; Fat: 10g; Protein: 10g; Carbs: 50g

Benefits: This colorful salad is a great way to get your daily veggies while enjoying a hearty meal rich in fiber and nutrients.

Cabbage and Carrot Slaw with Sesame Dressing

Benefits: This slaw is a crunchy, refreshing side dish that complements any meal, packed with vitamins and healthy fats from sesame oil.

Servings: 4
Preparation Time: 15 minutes
Cooking Time: 0 minutes

Ingredients:

- 4 cups shredded cabbage (green or purple)
- 2 cups shredded carrots
- 1/4 cup sesame oil
- 2 tablespoons apple cider vinegar
- 1 tablespoon honey or maple syrup (optional)
- Salt and pepper to taste

Instructions:

1. In a large bowl, combine shredded cabbage and carrots.
2. In a small bowl, whisk together sesame oil, apple cider vinegar, honey or maple syrup, salt, and pepper.
3. Pour the dressing over the slaw and toss to combine. Serve immediately or let it marinate in the refrigerator for an hour for better flavor.

Nutritional Information (per serving):

- Calories: 150; Fat: 14g; Protein: 2g; Carbs: 10g

Spaghetti Squash with Marinara Sauce

Benefits: This low-carb spaghetti alternative is a delicious way to enjoy your favorite pasta dish while staying aligned with the Good Energy diet.

Servings: 4
Preparation Time: 10 minutes
Cooking Time: 40 minutes

Ingredients:

- 1 medium spaghetti squash
- 2 cups marinara sauce (homemade or store-bought without additives)
- 2 tablespoons olive oil
- 1/4 cup fresh basil, chopped
- Salt and pepper to taste

Instructions:

1. Preheat the oven to 400°F (200°C). Cut the spaghetti squash in half and scoop out the seeds.
2. Brush with olive oil and season with salt and pepper. Place cut side down on a baking sheet and roast for 30-40 minutes until tender.
3. Once cooked, use a fork to scrape the insides into strands.
4. Heat marinara sauce in a saucepan and pour over the spaghetti squash strands.
5. Serve garnished with fresh basil.

Nutritional Information (per serving):

- Calories: 220; Fat: 10g; Protein: 5g; Carbs: 30g

Chapter 6 Dinner Recipes

Chapter 6 Dinner Recipes

Lemon Herb Grilled Chicken with Quinoa

Benefits: This dish is high in protein and healthy fats, providing a satisfying meal that supports muscle repair and overall energy levels.

Servings: 4
Preparation Time: 15 minutes
Cooking Time: 20 minutes

Ingredients:

- 4 boneless, skinless chicken breasts
- 1 cup quinoa
- 2 cups vegetable broth
- Juice of 1 lemon
- 2 tablespoons olive oil
- 2 garlic cloves, minced
- 1 tablespoon fresh thyme, chopped
- Salt and pepper to taste
- Fresh parsley for garnish

Instructions:

1. In a small bowl, mix lemon juice, olive oil, garlic, thyme, salt, and pepper. Marinate the chicken breasts in this mixture for at least 15 minutes.
2. While the chicken is marinating, rinse the quinoa under cold water. In a saucepan, combine quinoa and vegetable broth; bring to a boil.
3. Reduce heat, cover, and simmer for 15 minutes until the quinoa is fluffy and all the broth is absorbed.
4. Preheat a grill or grill pan over medium-high heat. Grill the marinated chicken for about 7-8 minutes per side, or until cooked through.
5. Serve the grilled chicken over a bed of quinoa, garnished with fresh parsley.

Nutritional Information (per serving):

- Calories: 350; Fat: 12g; Protein: 30g; Carbs: 35g

Vegetable Stir-Fry with Brown Rice

Benefits: This colorful stir-fry is rich in vitamins and minerals, offering a variety of textures and flavors while keeping your energy levels steady throughout the evening.

Servings: 4
Preparation Time: 15 minutes
Cooking Time: 15 minutes

Ingredients:

- 2 cups brown rice
- 4 cups mixed vegetables (broccoli, bell peppers, carrots, snap peas)
- 2 tablespoons olive oil
- 3 tablespoons low-sodium soy sauce (or tamari for gluten-free)
- 1 tablespoon ginger, minced
- 2 cloves garlic, minced
- Sesame seeds for garnish

Instructions:

1. Cook brown rice according to package instructions.
2. In a large skillet or wok, heat olive oil over medium-high heat. Add ginger and garlic; sauté for 1 minute until fragrant.
3. Add mixed vegetables and stir-fry for 5-7 minutes until tender-crisp.
4. Stir in the cooked brown rice and soy sauce, mixing well. Cook for an additional 2-3 minutes.
5. Serve hot, garnished with sesame seeds.

Nutritional Information (per serving):

- Calories: 280; Fat: 8g; Protein: 6g; Carbs: 46g

Baked Salmon with Asparagus

Benefits: This dish is rich in omega-3 fatty acids from the salmon, which support heart health, combined with the vitamins from asparagus, making it a nutritious and heart-friendly meal.

Servings: 4
Preparation Time: 10 minutes
Cooking Time: 20 minutes

Ingredients:

- 4 salmon fillets
- 1 bunch asparagus, trimmed
- 3 tablespoons olive oil
- Juice of 1 lemon
- 2 garlic cloves, minced
- Salt and pepper to taste

- Lemon wedges for serving

Instructions:

1. Preheat the oven to 400°F (200°C).
2. On a baking sheet, arrange the salmon fillets and asparagus. Drizzle with olive oil, lemon juice, garlic, salt, and pepper.
3. Bake for 15-20 minutes, or until the salmon is cooked through and flakes easily with a fork.
4. Serve with lemon wedges on the side.

Nutritional Information (per serving):

- Calories: 400; Fat: 25g; Protein: 35g; Carbs: 10g

Stuffed Bell Peppers with Quinoa and Turkey

Benefits: These stuffed peppers are a complete meal packed with protein and fiber, providing a satisfying option that keeps you full without weighing you down.

Servings: 4
Preparation Time: 15 minutes
Cooking Time: 30 minutes

Ingredients:

- 4 bell peppers, tops removed and seeds discarded
- 1 cup cooked quinoa
- 1 lb ground turkey (or plant-based alternative)
- 1 cup diced tomatoes (canned or fresh)
- 1 teaspoon Italian seasoning
- Salt and pepper to taste
- 1/2 cup shredded cheese (optional)

Instructions:

1. Preheat the oven to 375°F (190°C).
2. In a skillet, brown the ground turkey over medium heat. Add diced tomatoes, cooked quinoa, Italian seasoning, salt, and pepper; stir well.
3. Stuff each bell pepper with the turkey-quinoa mixture. If using cheese, sprinkle on top.
4. Place stuffed peppers in a baking dish, cover with foil, and bake for 25 minutes. Uncover and bake for an additional 5 minutes if cheese is used.
5. Serve warm.

Nutritional Information (per serving):

- Calories: 320; Fat: 10g; Protein: 30g; Carbs: 40g

Zucchini Noodles with Turkey Meatballs

Benefits: This dish offers a low-carb alternative to traditional spaghetti, while the turkey meatballs provide lean protein, making it a guilt-free and flavorful meal.

Servings: 4
Preparation Time: 20 minutes
Cooking Time: 20 minutes

Ingredients:

- 4 medium zucchinis, spiralized
- 1 lb ground turkey
- 1/4 cup grated Parmesan cheese (optional)
- 1 egg
- 1 teaspoon garlic powder
- 1 teaspoon Italian seasoning
- 2 cups marinara sauce (homemade or store-bought without additives)
- Olive oil for cooking

Instructions:

1. Preheat the oven to 400°F (200°C).
2. In a bowl, mix ground turkey, Parmesan cheese (if using), egg, garlic powder, and Italian seasoning. Form into meatballs.
3. Place meatballs on a baking sheet and bake for 15-20 minutes until cooked through.
4. In a skillet, heat olive oil over medium heat. Add spiralized zucchini and sauté for 3-5 minutes until just tender.
5. Serve zucchini noodles topped with marinara sauce and turkey meatballs.

Nutritional Information (per serving):

- Calories: 400; Fat: 15g; Protein: 35g; Carbs: 25g

Chickpea Curry with Brown Rice

Benefits: This comforting curry is rich in fiber and healthy fats, promoting digestive health while delivering a satisfying meal bursting with flavor.

Servings: 4
Preparation Time: 10 minutes
Cooking Time: 20 minutes

Ingredients:

- 1 can (15 oz) chickpeas, drained and rinsed
- 1 can (14 oz) coconut milk
- 1 cup diced tomatoes (canned or fresh)
- 1 onion, diced

- 2 tablespoons curry powder
- 2 cloves garlic, minced
- 1 tablespoon olive oil
- 2 cups brown rice

Instructions:

1. Cook brown rice according to package instructions.
2. In a large pot, heat olive oil over medium heat. Sauté onion and garlic until fragrant.
3. Add chickpeas, coconut milk, diced tomatoes, and curry powder; stir well.
4. Simmer for 15 minutes, allowing flavors to meld.
5. Serve over brown rice.

Nutritional Information (per serving):

- Calories: 350; Fat: 14g; Protein: 12g; Carbs: 45g

Spaghetti Squash with Roasted Vegetables

Benefits: This dish is a low-carb alternative that provides essential vitamins and minerals from the vegetables, making it a nutritious and satisfying dinner.

Servings: 4
Preparation Time: 15 minutes
Cooking Time: 40 minutes

Ingredients:

- 1 medium spaghetti squash
- 2 cups mixed vegetables (zucchini, bell peppers, carrots)
- 2 tablespoons olive oil
- 1 teaspoon Italian seasoning
- Salt and pepper to taste
- Fresh basil for garnish

Instructions:

1. Preheat the oven to 400°F (200°C).
2. Cut the spaghetti squash in half and scoop out the seeds. Brush with olive oil, salt, and pepper. Place cut side down on a baking sheet.
3. Toss mixed vegetables with olive oil, Italian seasoning, salt, and pepper. Spread on another baking sheet.
4. Bake both for 30-40 minutes until the squash is tender and vegetables are roasted.
5. Scrape the insides of the spaghetti squash into strands and mix with roasted vegetables. Garnish with fresh basil before serving.

Nutritional Information (per serving):

- Calories: 220; Fat: 8g; Protein: 4g; Carbs: 36g

Cilantro Lime Shrimp with Cauliflower Rice

Benefits: This dish is a fresh and zesty option high in protein, making it ideal for a light yet fulfilling dinner.

Servings: 4
Preparation Time: 10 minutes
Cooking Time: 10 minutes

Ingredients:

- 1 lb shrimp, peeled and deveined
- 2 cups cauliflower rice
- Juice of 2 limes
- 1/4 cup fresh cilantro, chopped
- 2 tablespoons olive oil
- 2 garlic cloves, minced
- Salt and pepper to taste

Instructions:

1. In a large skillet, heat olive oil over medium heat. Add garlic and shrimp; cook for 3-4 minutes until shrimp are pink.
2. Stir in lime juice, cilantro, salt, and pepper.
3. In a separate pan, sauté cauliflower rice in a bit of olive oil for about 5 minutes.
4. Serve the shrimp over cauliflower rice.

Nutritional Information (per serving):

- Calories: 280; Fat: 10g; Protein: 25g; Carbs: 15g

Sweet Potato and Black Bean Tacos

Benefits: These tacos are not only delicious but also packed with fiber and nutrients, keeping you satisfied while supporting healthy digestion.

Servings: 4
Preparation Time: 15 minutes
Cooking Time: 25 minutes

Ingredients:

- 2 medium sweet potatoes, diced
- 1 can (15 oz) black beans, drained and rinsed
- 1 teaspoon cumin
- 1 teaspoon chili powder
- 8 corn tortillas
- 1 avocado, sliced
- Fresh cilantro for garnish
- Lime wedges for serving

Instructions:

1. Preheat the oven to 400°F (200°C). Toss sweet pota-

toes with olive oil, cumin, chili powder, salt, and pepper. Roast for 20-25 minutes until tender.

2. In a saucepan, heat black beans until warm.

3. Warm corn tortillas in a dry skillet.

4. Assemble tacos with sweet potatoes, black beans, avocado slices, and garnish with cilantro. Serve with lime wedges.

Nutritional Information (per serving):
- Calories: 350; Fat: 12g; Protein: 10g; Carbs: 50g

Eggplant and Chickpea Stew

Benefits: This hearty stew is rich in plant-based protein and fiber, providing a warm and comforting meal that supports overall health.

Servings: 4
Preparation Time: 15 minutes
Cooking Time: 30 minutes

Ingredients:
- 1 large eggplant, diced
- 1 can (15 oz) chickpeas, drained and rinsed
- 1 can (14 oz) diced tomatoes
- 1 onion, diced
- 2 cloves garlic, minced
- 2 tablespoons olive oil
- 1 tablespoon cumin
- Salt and pepper to taste

Instructions:

1. In a large pot, heat olive oil over medium heat. Add onion and garlic; sauté until fragrant.

2. Stir in eggplant, chickpeas, diced tomatoes, cumin, salt, and pepper.

3. Simmer for 20-25 minutes until eggplant is tender.

4. Serve warm, garnished with fresh herbs if desired.

Nutritional Information (per serving):
- Calories: 280; Fat: 12g; Protein: 10g; Carbs: 35g

Grilled Portobello Mushrooms with Pesto

Benefits: This dish is low in calories but rich in flavor, providing healthy fats from the pesto and essential nutrients from mushrooms and tomatoes.

Servings: 4
Preparation Time: 10 minutes
Cooking Time: 15 minutes

Ingredients:
- 4 large portobello mushrooms
- 1/4 cup homemade or store-bought pesto (without additives)
- 1 cup cherry tomatoes, halved
- 2 tablespoons balsamic vinegar
- Olive oil for brushing
- Salt and pepper to taste

Instructions:

1. Preheat the grill to medium heat.

2. Brush portobello mushrooms with olive oil, and season with salt and pepper.

3. Grill for about 5-7 minutes on each side until tender.

4. In a bowl, toss cherry tomatoes with balsamic vinegar.

5. Serve grilled mushrooms topped with pesto and cherry tomatoes.

Nutritional Information (per serving):
- Calories: 200; Fat: 15g; Protein: 4g; Carbs: 10g

Oven-Baked Chicken Fajitas

Benefits: This meal is rich in protein and packed with colorful vegetables, providing a flavorful and nutritious option for your dinner table.

Servings: 4
Preparation Time: 15 minutes
Cooking Time: 30 minutes

Ingredients:
- 1 lb boneless, skinless chicken breasts, sliced
- 2 bell peppers, sliced
- 1 onion, sliced
- 2 tablespoons olive oil
- 2 teaspoons chili powder
- 1 teaspoon cumin
- Salt and pepper to taste
- Whole grain tortillas for serving

Instructions:

1. Preheat the oven to 425°F (220°C).

2. In a large bowl, combine chicken, bell peppers, onion, olive oil, chili powder, cumin, salt, and pepper.

3. Spread the mixture evenly on a baking sheet.

4. Bake for 25-30 minutes until chicken is cooked through and vegetables are tender.

5. Serve with whole grain tortillas.

Nutritional Information (per serving):
- Calories: 350; Fat: 10g; Protein: 30g; Carbs: 30g

Cauliflower and Chickpea Salad

Benefits: This salad is a fantastic source of protein and fiber, providing a satisfying yet light dinner option that supports digestive health.

Servings: 4
Preparation Time: 15 minutes
Cooking Time: 15 minutes

Ingredients:

- 1 head cauliflower, cut into florets
- 1 can (15 oz) chickpeas, drained and rinsed
- 1/4 cup olive oil
- 2 tablespoons apple cider vinegar
- 1 teaspoon cumin
- Salt and pepper to taste
- Fresh parsley for garnish

Instructions:

1. Preheat the oven to 400°F (200°C).
2. Toss cauliflower florets with olive oil, cumin, salt, and pepper. Roast for 15 minutes until tender.
3. In a large bowl, combine roasted cauliflower, chickpeas, and apple cider vinegar.
4. Toss well and garnish with fresh parsley before serving.

Nutritional Information (per serving):

- Calories: 250; Fat: 12g; Protein: 10g; Carbs: 30g

Baked Cod with Lemon and Garlic

Benefits: This dish is rich in protein and low in carbs, providing a light yet filling dinner that supports muscle health and overall well-being.

Servings: 4
Preparation Time: 10 minutes
Cooking Time: 20 minutes

Ingredients:

- 4 cod fillets
- 3 tablespoons olive oil
- Juice of 1 lemon
- 4 garlic cloves, minced
- Salt and pepper to taste
- Fresh parsley for garnish

Instructions:

1. Preheat the oven to 375°F (190°C).
2. Place cod fillets in a baking dish. In a bowl, mix olive oil, lemon juice, garlic, salt, and pepper; pour over the fish.

3. Bake for 15-20 minutes until the fish flakes easily with a fork.
4. Serve garnished with fresh parsley.

Nutritional Information (per serving):

- Calories: 280; Fat: 15g; Protein: 30g; Carbs: 5g

Moroccan Lentil Stew

Benefits: This stew is hearty and filling, packed with plant-based protein and fiber, making it an excellent choice for a nutritious dinner.

Servings: 4
Preparation Time: 15 minutes
Cooking Time: 30 minutes

Ingredients:

- 1 cup lentils, rinsed
- 1 onion, diced
- 2 carrots, diced
- 2 cloves garlic, minced
- 1 can (14 oz) diced tomatoes
- 2 teaspoons cumin
- 1 teaspoon cinnamon
- 4 cups vegetable broth
- Salt and pepper to taste
- Fresh cilantro for garnish

Instructions:

1. In a large pot, heat olive oil over medium heat. Sauté onion and garlic until fragrant.
2. Add carrots, lentils, diced tomatoes, cumin, cinnamon, salt, and pepper. Stir well.
3. Pour in vegetable broth and bring to a boil. Reduce heat and simmer for 25-30 minutes until lentils are tender.
4. Serve warm, garnished with fresh cilantro.

Nutritional Information (per serving):

- Calories: 300; Fat: 6g; Protein: 15g; Carbs: 50g

Chapter 7 Beef Recipes

Chapter 7 Beef Recipes

Grilled Lemon Herb Beef Skewers

Benefits: These skewers are packed with lean protein and healthy fats, making them a satisfying meal that supports muscle recovery and provides essential nutrients for overall energy.

Servings: 4
Preparation Time: 15 minutes
Cooking Time: 10 minutes

Ingredients:

- 1 lb beef sirloin, cut into 1-inch cubes
- 1/4 cup olive oil
- Juice of 2 lemons
- 2 garlic cloves, minced
- 1 tablespoon fresh rosemary, chopped
- 1 tablespoon fresh thyme, chopped
- Salt and pepper to taste
- 1 red onion, cut into wedges
- 1 bell pepper, cut into chunks

Instructions:

1. In a bowl, mix olive oil, lemon juice, garlic, rosemary, thyme, salt, and pepper to create a marinade.
2. Add beef cubes to the marinade and let sit for at least 30 minutes.
3. Preheat the grill to medium-high heat.
4. Thread beef, onion, and bell pepper onto skewers.
5. Grill skewers for about 8-10 minutes, turning occasionally, until beef is cooked to desired doneness.
6. Serve hot, garnished with fresh herbs if desired.

Nutritional Information (per serving):

- Calories: 320; Fat: 20g; Protein: 30g; Carbs: 5g

Slow Cooker Beef and Vegetable Stew

Benefits: This hearty stew is rich in protein and fiber, providing a wholesome meal that warms the soul and fuels the body, perfect for a chilly evening.

Servings: 6
Preparation Time: 15 minutes
Cooking Time: 6 hours

Ingredients:

- 2 lbs beef chuck, cut into 1-inch cubes
- 4 cups beef broth (low sodium)
- 4 carrots, sliced
- 3 potatoes, diced
- 2 stalks celery, chopped
- 1 onion, diced
- 2 cloves garlic, minced
- 1 tablespoon fresh thyme, chopped
- 1 tablespoon fresh parsley, chopped
- Salt and pepper to taste

Instructions:

1. In a slow cooker, combine beef, broth, carrots, potatoes, celery, onion, garlic, thyme, salt, and pepper.
2. Stir well to mix all ingredients.
3. Cover and cook on low for 6-8 hours, or until beef is tender.
4. Before serving, stir in fresh parsley.

Nutritional Information (per serving):

- Calories: 350; Fat: 15g; Protein: 30g; Carbs: 35g

Spicy Beef and Broccoli Stir-Fry

Benefits: This quick stir-fry is loaded with vitamins and minerals from broccoli while providing a spicy kick, making it a delicious way to enjoy lean protein.

Servings: 4

Preparation Time: 15 minutes

Cooking Time: 10 minutes

Ingredients:

- 1 lb flank steak, sliced thinly against the grain
- 4 cups broccoli florets
- 2 tablespoons olive oil
- 3 cloves garlic, minced
- 2 tablespoons low-sodium soy sauce (or tamari)
- 1 tablespoon red pepper flakes (adjust to taste)
- 1 teaspoon ginger, minced
- Salt and pepper to taste

Instructions:

1. Heat olive oil in a large skillet or wok over medium-high heat.
2. Add garlic and ginger; sauté for 1 minute until fragrant.
3. Add the sliced flank steak and cook for 3-4 minutes until browned.
4. Add broccoli and stir-fry for another 3-4 minutes.
5. Pour in soy sauce and red pepper flakes, mixing well.
6. Serve hot, over brown rice or quinoa if desired.

Nutritional Information (per serving):

- Calories: 300; Fat: 15g; Protein: 30g; Carbs: 10g

Beef and Quinoa Stuffed Peppers

Benefits: These stuffed peppers are a nutrient-dense meal rich in protein and fiber, making them an excellent option for a filling dinner without unnecessary carbs.

Servings: 4

Preparation Time: 15 minutes

Cooking Time: 30 minutes

Ingredients:

- 4 large bell peppers, tops cut off and seeds removed
- 1 lb ground beef (grass-fed if possible)
- 1 cup cooked quinoa
- 1 can (15 oz) diced tomatoes
- 1 tablespoon Italian seasoning
- Salt and pepper to taste
- 1 cup shredded cheese (optional)

Instructions:

1. Preheat the oven to 375°F (190°C).
2. In a skillet, brown the ground beef over medium heat. Add diced tomatoes, cooked quinoa, Italian seasoning, salt, and pepper; stir to combine.
3. Stuff each bell pepper with the beef and quinoa mixture. If desired, top with cheese.
4. Place stuffed peppers in a baking dish and cover with foil. Bake for 25-30 minutes.
5. Serve warm.

Nutritional Information (per serving):

- Calories: 400; Fat: 20g; Protein: 30g; Carbs: 30g

Beef and Sweet Potato Hash

Benefits: This savory hash combines the sweetness of sweet potatoes with the richness of beef, providing a balanced meal that is perfect for breakfast, lunch, or dinner.

Servings: 4

Preparation Time: 15 minutes

Cooking Time: 20 minutes

Ingredients:

- 1 lb ground beef (lean)
- 2 medium sweet potatoes, diced
- 1 onion, diced
- 2 cloves garlic, minced
- 2 tablespoons olive oil
- 1 teaspoon smoked paprika
- Salt and pepper to taste
- Fresh parsley for garnish

Instructions:

1. Heat olive oil in a large skillet over medium heat.
2. Add diced sweet potatoes and cook for 10 minutes until slightly tender.
3. Stir in onion and garlic; cook for another 5 minutes.
4. Add ground beef, smoked paprika, salt, and pepper. Cook until beef is browned and sweet potatoes are fully tender.

5. Garnish with fresh parsley before serving.

Nutritional Information (per serving):

- Calories: 400; Fat: 22g; Protein: 25g; Carbs: 30g

Classic Beef Tacos with Avocado Salsa

Benefits: These tacos offer a healthy twist on a classic favorite, featuring lean beef and fresh ingredients, making them a satisfying meal that's also easy to prepare.

Servings: 4
Preparation Time: 15 minutes
Cooking Time: 10 minutes

Ingredients:

- 1 lb ground beef (lean)
- 1 tablespoon taco seasoning (homemade or store-bought without additives)
- 8 corn tortillas
- 1 avocado, diced
- 1/2 cup diced tomatoes
- 1/4 cup chopped red onion
- Fresh cilantro for garnish
- Lime wedges for serving

Instructions:

1. In a skillet, cook ground beef over medium heat until browned. Add taco seasoning and a splash of water; stir to combine.
2. Warm corn tortillas in a dry skillet.
3. Assemble tacos with seasoned beef and top with avocado salsa (mix avocado, tomatoes, onion, and cilantro).
4. Serve with lime wedges on the side.

Nutritional Information (per serving):

- Calories: 350; Fat: 20g; Protein: 25g; Carbs: 20g

Beef and Mushroom Stir-Fry

Benefits: This stir-fry is not only quick to make but also packed with nutrients, combining lean protein from beef with fiber-rich vegetables for a balanced meal.

Servings: 4
Preparation Time: 15 minutes
Cooking Time: 10 minutes

Ingredients:

- 1 lb beef sirloin, sliced thinly
- 2 cups mushrooms, sliced
- 1 bell pepper, sliced
- 2 tablespoons olive oil
- 3 cloves garlic, minced
- 2 tablespoons low-sodium soy sauce (or tamari)
- 1 teaspoon ginger, minced
- Salt and pepper to taste

Instructions:

1. Heat olive oil in a skillet over medium-high heat. Add garlic and ginger; sauté for 1 minute.
2. Add sliced beef and cook until browned.
3. Stir in mushrooms and bell pepper; cook for an additional 3-4 minutes.
4. Add soy sauce, salt, and pepper; stir well.
5. Serve over brown rice or quinoa if desired.

Nutritional Information (per serving):

- Calories: 320; Fat: 15g; Protein: 30g; Carbs: 10g

Beef Lettuce Wraps

Benefits: These lettuce wraps are a fresh and light alternative to traditional tacos, offering a delicious way to enjoy lean protein while keeping carbs to a minimum.

Servings: 4
Preparation Time: 15 minutes
Cooking Time: 10 minutes

Ingredients:

- 1 lb ground beef (lean)
- 1 cup diced bell peppers
- 1/2 cup diced onions
- 3 cloves garlic, minced
- 2 tablespoons low-sodium soy sauce (or tamari)
- 1 tablespoon sesame oil
- Salt and pepper to taste
- Butter or romaine lettuce leaves for wrapping
- Sliced green onions for garnish

Instructions:

1. In a skillet, heat sesame oil over medium heat. Add onions and garlic; sauté until fragrant.

2. Add ground beef and cook until browned.

3. Stir in bell peppers, soy sauce, salt, and pepper; cook for an additional 3-4 minutes.

4. Serve the beef mixture in lettuce leaves and garnish with green onions.

Nutritional Information (per serving):

- Calories: 300; Fat: 18g; Protein: 25g; Carbs: 5g

Teriyaki Beef Bowl

Benefits: This teriyaki bowl provides a balanced meal with protein, healthy fats, and fiber-rich vegetables, making it a nutritious option for lunch or dinner.

Servings: 4

Preparation Time: 15 minutes

Cooking Time: 15 minutes

Ingredients:

- 1 lb flank steak, sliced thinly
- 1/4 cup low-sodium soy sauce (or tamari)
- 2 tablespoons honey (or maple syrup)
- 1 tablespoon sesame oil
- 2 cups steamed broccoli
- 2 cups cooked brown rice
- 1 tablespoon sesame seeds for garnish
- Sliced green onions for garnish

Instructions:

1. In a bowl, mix soy sauce, honey, and sesame oil. Add the sliced flank steak and marinate for at least 15 minutes.

2. Heat a skillet over medium-high heat; cook marinated beef until browned, about 5-7 minutes.

3. Serve beef over steamed broccoli and brown rice, garnished with sesame seeds and green onions.

Nutritional Information (per serving):

- Calories: 450; Fat: 15g; Protein: 30g; Carbs: 50g

Beef and Spinach Stuffed Mushrooms

Benefits: These stuffed mushrooms are a low-carb option that delivers a satisfying punch of flavor and nutrients, combining protein with the goodness of leafy greens.

Servings: 4

Preparation Time: 15 minutes

Cooking Time: 20 minutes

Ingredients:

- 1 lb ground beef (lean)
- 12 large portobello mushrooms, stems removed
- 2 cups fresh spinach, chopped
- 1/2 cup onion, diced
- 3 cloves garlic, minced
- 1/4 cup Parmesan cheese, grated (optional)
- 2 tablespoons olive oil
- Salt and pepper to taste

Instructions:

1. Preheat the oven to 375°F (190°C).

2. In a skillet, heat olive oil over medium heat. Sauté onion and garlic until fragrant.

3. Add ground beef and cook until browned. Stir in chopped spinach, salt, and pepper; cook until spinach wilts.

4. Spoon the beef mixture into portobello mushrooms. If desired, sprinkle with Parmesan cheese.

5. Place stuffed mushrooms on a baking sheet and bake for 15-20 minutes.

Nutritional Information (per serving):

- Calories: 300; Fat: 18g; Protein: 25g; Carbs: 8g

Beef and Zucchini Noodles

Benefits: This dish replaces traditional pasta with nutrient-dense zucchini noodles, offering a delicious and low-carb meal that is rich in protein and flavor.

Servings: 4

Preparation Time: 15 minutes

Cooking Time: 10 minutes

Ingredients:

- 1 lb ground beef (lean)

- 4 medium zucchinis, spiralized
- 1 cup cherry tomatoes, halved
- 3 cloves garlic, minced
- 2 tablespoons olive oil
- 1 teaspoon Italian seasoning
- Salt and pepper to taste

Instructions:

1. In a large skillet, heat olive oil over medium heat. Add garlic and sauté for 1 minute.

2. Add ground beef and cook until browned.

3. Stir in cherry tomatoes, Italian seasoning, salt, and pepper; cook for 3-4 minutes.

4. Add spiralized zucchini noodles and cook for an additional 2-3 minutes until tender.

5. Serve hot, garnished with fresh herbs if desired.

Nutritional Information (per serving):

Benefits: These stuffed mushrooms are a low-carb option that delivers a satisfying punch of flavor and nutrients, combining protein with the goodness of leafy greens.

- Calories: 350; Fat: 20g; Protein: 30g; Carbs: 10g

Beef and Bell Pepper Stir-Fry

Benefits: This quick and colorful stir-fry is a great way to incorporate fresh vegetables into your diet while enjoying a lean protein source.

Servings: 4
Preparation Time: 15 minutes
Cooking Time: 10 minutes

Ingredients:

- 1 lb beef sirloin, sliced thinly
- 2 bell peppers, sliced
- 1 onion, sliced
- 2 tablespoons olive oil
- 2 tablespoons low-sodium soy sauce (or tamari)
- 1 teaspoon ginger, minced
- Salt and pepper to taste

Instructions:

1. Heat olive oil in a skillet over medium-high heat. Add sliced beef and cook until browned.

2. Add bell peppers, onion, ginger, salt, and pepper; stir-fry for 3-4 minutes until vegetables are tender.

3. Pour in soy sauce and mix well.

4. Serve hot, over brown rice or quinoa if desired.

Nutritional Information (per serving):

- Calories: 300; Fat: 15g; Protein: 30g; Carbs: 10g

Beef and Cabbage Skillet

Benefits: This skillet dish combines protein-rich beef with fiber-packed cabbage, making it a filling meal that supports digestion and overall health.

Servings: 4
Preparation Time: 15 minutes
Cooking Time: 15 minutes

Ingredients:

- 1 lb ground beef (lean)
- 1/2 head cabbage, chopped
- 1 onion, diced
- 2 cloves garlic, minced
- 2 tablespoons olive oil
- 1 teaspoon paprika
- Salt and pepper to taste

Instructions:

1. In a large skillet, heat olive oil over medium heat. Add onion and garlic; sauté until fragrant.

2. Add ground beef and cook until browned.

3. Stir in chopped cabbage, paprika, salt, and pepper; cook for another 5-7 minutes until cabbage is tender.

4. Serve warm.

Nutritional Information (per serving):

- Calories: 300; Fat: 20g; Protein: 25g; Carbs: 10g

Herbed Beef and Carrot Soup

Benefits: This comforting soup is a great source of protein and vitamins, making it a nourishing choice for cold days or whenever you need a cozy meal.

Servings: 4
Preparation Time: 15 minutes
Cooking Time: 30 minutes

Ingredients:

- 1 lb beef stew meat, cubed
- 4 cups beef broth (low sodium)
- 3 carrots, sliced
- 1 onion, diced
- 2 cloves garlic, minced
- 1 tablespoon fresh thyme, chopped
- 1 tablespoon fresh parsley, chopped
- Salt and pepper to taste

Instructions:

1. In a large pot, brown the beef over medium heat.
2. Add onions and garlic; sauté until fragrant.
3. Pour in beef broth and bring to a boil. Add carrots, thyme, salt, and pepper.
4. Reduce heat and simmer for 25-30 minutes until beef is tender.
5. Stir in fresh parsley before serving.

Nutritional Information (per serving):

- Calories: 350; Fat: 15g; Protein: 30g; Carbs: 20g

Beef and Cauliflower Rice Bowl

Benefits: This bowl offers a low-carb alternative to rice, packed with nutrients and protein, making it a perfect option for a healthy and satisfying meal.

Servings: 4
Preparation Time: 15 minutes
Cooking Time: 10 minutes

Ingredients:

- 1 lb ground beef (lean)
- 1 head cauliflower, grated into rice
- 1 cup diced bell peppers
- 2 cloves garlic, minced
- 2 tablespoons olive oil
- 2 tablespoons low-sodium soy sauce (or tamari)
- Salt and pepper to taste

Instructions:

1. In a large skillet, heat olive oil over medium heat. Add garlic and sauté for 1 minute.
2. Add ground beef and cook until browned.
3. Stir in grated cauliflower and bell peppers; cook for 5-7 minutes.
4. Add soy sauce, salt, and pepper; mix well.
5. Serve hot, garnished with fresh herbs if desired.

Nutritional Information (per serving):

- Calories: 300; Fat: 18g; Protein: 25g; Carbs: 10g

Chapter 8 Poultry Recipes

Chapter 8 Poultry Recipes

Lemon Herb Grilled Chicken

Benefits: This Lemon Herb Grilled Chicken is a perfect option for a quick and healthy dinner. The marinade adds a burst of flavor while the lean protein helps maintain muscle mass and promote satiety.

Servings: 4
Preparation Time: 15 minutes
Cooking Time: 20 minutes

Ingredients:

- 4 boneless, skinless chicken breasts
- 1/4 cup olive oil
- Juice of 2 lemons
- Zest of 1 lemon
- 2 cloves garlic, minced
- 1 tablespoon fresh rosemary, chopped
- 1 tablespoon fresh thyme, chopped
- Salt and pepper to taste

Instructions:

1. In a mixing bowl, combine olive oil, lemon juice, lemon zest, garlic, rosemary, thyme, salt, and pepper. Whisk until well mixed.
2. Place chicken breasts in a resealable plastic bag and pour the marinade over the chicken. Seal the bag and refrigerate for at least 30 minutes, preferably overnight.
3. Preheat the grill to medium-high heat. Remove chicken from marinade and discard the leftover marinade.
4. Grill chicken for about 6-7 minutes on each side or until fully cooked and juices run clear.
5. Serve with a side of grilled vegetables for a complete meal.

Nutritional Information:

- Calories: 280; Fat: 12g; Protein: 34g; Carbs: 2g

Spicy Chicken Stir-Fry

Benefits: This Spicy Chicken Stir-Fry is packed with colorful vegetables and protein. The ginger and red pepper flakes not only enhance flavor but also provide anti-inflammatory benefits.

Servings: 4
Preparation Time: 10 minutes
Cooking Time: 15 minutes

Ingredients:

- 1 pound chicken breast, sliced thinly
- 2 tablespoons coconut oil
- 1 bell pepper, sliced
- 1 cup broccoli florets
- 1 cup snap peas
- 2 tablespoons low-sodium soy sauce
- 1 tablespoon fresh ginger, grated
- 2 cloves garlic, minced
- 1 teaspoon red pepper flakes

Instructions:

1. Heat coconut oil in a large skillet over medium-high heat. Add sliced chicken and cook until browned and cooked through, about 5-7 minutes.
2. Add bell pepper, broccoli, and snap peas to the skillet. Stir-fry for another 5 minutes until vegetables are tender-crisp.
3. In a small bowl, mix soy sauce, ginger, garlic, and red pepper flakes. Pour over the chicken and vegetables, stirring to coat evenly.
4. Cook for an additional 2-3 minutes. Serve hot.

Nutritional Information:

- Calories: 320; Fat: 16g; Protein: 28g; Carbs: 22g

Chicken and Quinoa Bowl

Benefits: The Chicken and Quinoa Bowl is a wholesome meal that provides a complete protein source. Quinoa is a fantastic gluten-free grain high in protein and fiber, making it ideal for energy and digestion.

Servings: 4
Preparation Time: 15 minutes
Cooking Time: 25 minutes

Ingredients:

- 1 pound chicken breast, diced
- 1 cup quinoa
- 2 cups vegetable broth
- 1 cup spinach, chopped
- 1 bell pepper, diced
- 1/4 cup cilantro, chopped
- 1 tablespoon olive oil
- 1 teaspoon cumin
- Salt and pepper to taste

Instructions:

1. Rinse quinoa under cold water. In a medium saucepan, bring vegetable broth to a boil and add quinoa. Reduce heat, cover, and simmer for 15 minutes or until liquid is absorbed.
2. In a large skillet, heat olive oil over medium heat. Add diced chicken and cook until golden brown and cooked through, about 7-10 minutes.
3. Add bell pepper and spinach to the skillet, cooking until spinach is wilted.
4. Stir in cooked quinoa, cumin, cilantro, salt, and pepper. Mix well and serve warm.

Nutritional Information:

- Calories: 350; Fat: 9g; Protein: 32g; Carbs: 42g

Coconut Curry Chicken

Benefits: This Coconut Curry Chicken is a delightful dish that offers rich flavors and creamy texture without any heavy creams. The curry powder adds not just taste but also aids in digestion and boosts immunity.

Servings: 4
Preparation Time: 15 minutes
Cooking Time: 25 minutes

Ingredients:

- 1 pound chicken breast, cubed
- 1 can (14 oz) coconut milk
- 2 tablespoons curry powder
- 1 onion, diced
- 2 cloves garlic, minced
- 1 tablespoon olive oil
- 1 cup cauliflower florets
- 1 cup green beans, trimmed
- Salt and pepper to taste

Instructions:

1. Heat olive oil in a large skillet over medium heat. Add onion and garlic, sautéing until softened.
2. Add cubed chicken and cook until browned on all sides.
3. Stir in curry powder, then add coconut milk, cauliflower, and green beans.
4. Bring to a simmer and cook for about 15 minutes, or until vegetables are tender and chicken is cooked through.
5. Season with salt and pepper, and serve warm.

Nutritional Information:

- Calories: 370; Fat: 24g; Protein: 28g; Carbs: 12g

Baked Honey Mustard Chicken Thighs

Benefits: These Baked Honey Mustard Chicken Thighs offer a sweet and tangy flavor profile. The use of raw honey provides natural sweetness and antioxidants, making this dish not only tasty but also health-conscious.

Servings: 4
Preparation Time: 10 minutes
Cooking Time: 35 minutes

Ingredients:
- 4 bone-in, skin-on chicken thighs
- 1/4 cup Dijon mustard
- 1/4 cup raw honey
- 2 cloves garlic, minced
- 1 tablespoon apple cider vinegar
- Salt and pepper to taste

Instructions:
1. Preheat the oven to 375°F (190°C).
2. In a small bowl, whisk together Dijon mustard, honey, garlic, apple cider vinegar, salt, and pepper.
3. Place chicken thighs in a baking dish and pour the honey mustard mixture over them, coating evenly.
4. Bake for 30-35 minutes or until chicken is cooked through and juices run clear.
5. Let rest for 5 minutes before serving.

Nutritional Information:
- Calories: 400; Fat: 25g; Protein: 30g; Carbs: 14g

Mediterranean Chicken Salad

Benefits: This Mediterranean Chicken Salad is a nutrient-dense option filled with vegetables and healthy fats. The variety of colors and textures not only makes it appealing but also supports a balanced diet rich in vitamins and minerals.

Servings: 4
Preparation Time: 15 minutes
Cooking Time: 20 minutes

Ingredients:
- 1 pound grilled chicken breast, diced
- 2 cups mixed greens
- 1 cup cherry tomatoes, halved
- 1/2 cucumber, diced
- 1/4 red onion, thinly sliced
- 1/4 cup olives, sliced
- 1/4 cup feta cheese, crumbled
- 1/4 cup olive oil
- 2 tablespoons red wine vinegar
- Salt and pepper to taste

Instructions:
1. In a large bowl, combine mixed greens, cherry tomatoes, cucumber, red onion, olives, and feta cheese.
2. Add diced grilled chicken on top.
3. In a small bowl, whisk together olive oil, red wine vinegar, salt, and pepper.
4. Drizzle the dressing over the salad and toss gently to combine.
5. Serve immediately for a refreshing meal.

Nutritional Information:
- Calories: 320; Fat: 22g; Protein: 28g; Carbs: 12g

Garlic Herb Roasted Chicken

Benefits: This Garlic Herb Roasted Chicken is full of flavor and makes a stunning centerpiece for any meal. The herbs not only enhance taste but also provide various health benefits, including anti-inflammatory properties.

Servings: 6
Preparation Time: 10 minutes
Cooking Time: 1 hour

Ingredients:
- 1 whole chicken (about 4-5 pounds)
- 1/4 cup olive oil
- 4 cloves garlic, minced
- 1 tablespoon fresh thyme, chopped
- 1 tablespoon fresh rosemary, chopped
- 1 tablespoon lemon juice
- Salt and pepper to taste

Instructions:
1. Preheat the oven to 425°F (220°C).
2. In a small bowl, mix olive oil, garlic, thyme, rosemary, lemon juice, salt, and pepper.
3. Place the chicken in a roasting pan and rub the herb mixture all over the chicken, including under the skin.
4. Roast in the oven for about 1 hour or until the internal temperature reaches 165°F (75°C).
5. Let rest for 10 minutes before carving.

Nutritional Information:
- Calories: 480; Fat: 28g; Protein: 45g; Carbs: 0g

Chicken and Vegetable Skewers

Benefits: These Chicken and Vegetable Skewers are a fun and interactive way to enjoy a meal. The mix of colorful vegetables provides a variety of nutrients, making this dish as healthy as it is delicious.

Servings: 4
Preparation Time: 15 minutes
Cooking Time: 10 minutes

Ingredients:

- 1 pound chicken breast, cubed
- 1 zucchini, sliced
- 1 bell pepper, chopped
- 1 red onion, chopped
- 1 cup cherry tomatoes
- 2 tablespoons olive oil
- 1 tablespoon Italian seasoning
- Salt and pepper to taste

Instructions:

1. Preheat the grill to medium heat.
2. In a bowl, combine olive oil, Italian seasoning, salt, and pepper. Add chicken and vegetables, tossing to coat.
3. Thread chicken and vegetables onto skewers alternately.
4. Grill skewers for about 10 minutes, turning occasionally until chicken is cooked through.
5. Serve with a side of quinoa or brown rice.

Nutritional Information:

- Calories: 280; Fat: 12g; Protein: 30g; Carbs: 8g

Chicken and Spinach Stuffed Peppers

Benefits: These Chicken and Spinach Stuffed Peppers are nutrient-packed and visually appealing. They are a fantastic way to incorporate more vegetables into your diet while providing a filling and satisfying meal.

Servings: 4
Preparation Time: 20 minutes
Cooking Time: 30 minutes

Ingredients:

- 4 bell peppers (any color)
- 1 pound ground chicken
- 2 cups spinach, chopped
- 1 cup cooked brown rice
- 1 teaspoon garlic powder
- 1 teaspoon onion powder
- Salt and pepper to taste
- 1 cup diced tomatoes (canned or fresh)

Instructions:

1. Preheat the oven to 375°F (190°C). Cut the tops off the bell peppers and remove seeds.
2. In a skillet over medium heat, cook ground chicken until browned. Add spinach, cooked rice, garlic powder, onion powder, salt, pepper, and tomatoes. Stir until spinach wilts.
3. Stuff each bell pepper with the chicken mixture. Place in a baking dish and cover with foil.
4. Bake for 25-30 minutes until peppers are tender.
5. Serve warm.

Nutritional Information:

- Calories: 320; Fat: 10g; Protein: 28g; Carbs: 36g

Cilantro Lime Chicken Tacos

Benefits: These Cilantro Lime Chicken Tacos are refreshing and zesty. The use of corn tortillas provides a gluten-free option that pairs beautifully with the marinated chicken, making it a satisfying meal.

Servings: 4
Preparation Time: 15 minutes
Cooking Time: 15 minutes

Ingredients:

- 1 pound chicken breast, sliced thin
- 1/4 cup lime juice
- 1/4 cup cilantro, chopped
- 1 teaspoon cumin
- 1 teaspoon paprika
- Salt and pepper to taste
- Corn tortillas (for serving)
- Optional toppings: avocado, salsa, lettuce

Instructions:

1. In a bowl, combine lime juice, cilantro, cumin, paprika, salt, and pepper. Add sliced chicken and marinate for at least 15 minutes.
2. Heat a skillet over medium-high heat and cook marinated chicken until fully cooked, about 5-7 minutes.
3. Warm corn tortillas in a separate pan or microwave.
4. Assemble tacos by placing chicken on tortillas and adding desired toppings.
5. Serve with lime wedges for extra flavor.

Nutritional Information:

- Calories: 350; Fat: 10g; Protein: 30g; Carbs: 40g

Chicken Cacciatore

Benefits: This Chicken Cacciatore is a hearty dish that brings classic Italian flavors to your table. The combination of chicken with vegetables creates a rich, satisfying meal packed with nutrients.

Servings: 4
Preparation Time: 15 minutes
Cooking Time: 45 minutes

Ingredients:

- 1 pound chicken thighs, bone-in
- 1 onion, sliced
- 2 bell peppers, sliced
- 2 cloves garlic, minced
- 1 can (14 oz) diced tomatoes
- 1 teaspoon oregano
- 1 teaspoon basil
- Salt and pepper to taste
- 1 tablespoon olive oil

Instructions:

1. In a large skillet, heat olive oil over medium heat. Add chicken thighs and brown on all sides, about 10 minutes.
2. Remove chicken and add onion, bell peppers, and garlic to the skillet. Sauté until softened.
3. Return chicken to the skillet, add diced tomatoes, oregano, basil, salt, and pepper.
4. Simmer for 30 minutes, covered, until chicken is cooked through and tender.
5. Serve over whole grain pasta or brown rice.

Nutritional Information:

- Calories: 400; Fat: 22g; Protein: 35g; Carbs: 12g

BBQ Chicken Lettuce Wraps

Benefits: These BBQ Chicken Lettuce Wraps are a fun and low-carb alternative to traditional tacos. They are perfect for a quick meal or appetizer and provide a satisfying crunch with every bite.

Servings: 4
Preparation Time: 15 minutes
Cooking Time: 15 minutes

Ingredients:

- 1 pound shredded cooked chicken
- 1/2 cup homemade BBQ sauce (no refined sugar)
- 1 head of butter lettuce, leaves separated
- 1 carrot, shredded
- 1/2 cucumber, diced
- Green onions, sliced (for garnish)

Instructions:

1. In a bowl, mix shredded chicken with BBQ sauce until well coated.
2. In a large skillet over medium heat, warm the BBQ chicken for about 5 minutes.
3. To assemble, take a lettuce leaf and fill it with BBQ chicken, shredded carrot, and cucumber.
4. Garnish with sliced green onions and serve immediately.

Nutritional Information:

- Calories: 250; Fat: 10g; Protein: 28g; Carbs: 10g

Orange Ginger Chicken Stir-Fry

Benefits: This Orange Ginger Chicken Stir-Fry is vibrant and full of flavor. The citrus not only brightens the dish but also provides vitamin C, making it a great immune-boosting meal.

Servings: 4
Preparation Time: 15 minutes
Cooking Time: 10 minutes

Ingredients:

- 1 pound chicken breast, thinly sliced
- 2 tablespoons olive oil
- 1 cup broccoli florets
- 1 bell pepper, sliced
- 1 carrot, julienned
- Juice and zest of 1 orange
- 1 tablespoon fresh ginger, grated
- Salt and pepper to taste

Instructions:

1. Heat olive oil in a large skillet over medium-high heat. Add chicken slices and cook until no longer pink, about 5-7 minutes.
2. Add broccoli, bell pepper, and carrot to the skillet. Stir-fry for another 3-4 minutes.
3. Add orange juice, zest, ginger, salt, and pepper. Stir to combine and cook for an additional 2 minutes.
4. Serve hot over brown rice or quinoa.

Nutritional Information:

- Calories: 300; Fat: 10g; Protein: 30g; Carbs: 20g

Chicken Piccata

Benefits: Chicken Piccata is a light and flavorful dish that showcases the tanginess of lemon and capers. It's a great way to enjoy a classic Italian dish with a healthier twist.

Servings: 4
Preparation Time: 15 minutes
Cooking Time: 20 minutes

Ingredients:

- 1 pound chicken breasts, pounded thin
- 1/4 cup coconut flour (for dredging)
- 3 tablespoons olive oil
- 2 tablespoons capers, rinsed
- Juice of 1 lemon
- 1/2 cup chicken broth (low-sodium)
- Fresh parsley, chopped (for garnish)

Instructions:

1. Dredge chicken breasts in coconut flour, shaking off excess.
2. In a skillet, heat olive oil over medium heat. Add chicken and cook until golden brown, about 5 minutes per side.
3. Remove chicken from skillet and set aside.
4. In the same skillet, add capers, lemon juice, and chicken broth, scraping the bottom of the pan to deglaze.
5. Return chicken to the skillet, simmering for 5 minutes to absorb flavors.
6. Garnish with parsley and serve.

Nutritional Information:

- Calories: 320; Fat: 16g; Protein: 32g; Carbs: 6g

Teriyaki Chicken Bowls

Benefits: These Teriyaki Chicken Bowls are a deliciously satisfying meal that offers a balance of protein, fiber, and healthy carbs. The homemade teriyaki sauce is a healthier alternative, making this dish perfect for the Good Energy diet.

Servings: 4
Preparation Time: 15 minutes
Cooking Time: 20 minutes

Ingredients:

- 1 pound chicken breast, diced
- 1/4 cup low-sodium soy sauce
- 2 tablespoons honey
- 1 tablespoon sesame oil
- 1 teaspoon garlic powder
- 1 cup brown rice
- 1 cup mixed vegetables (carrots, bell peppers, broccoli)

Instructions:

1. Cook brown rice according to package instructions.
2. In a bowl, mix soy sauce, honey, sesame oil, and garlic powder.
3. In a skillet over medium heat, add diced chicken and cook until browned.
4. Pour the sauce over the chicken and add mixed vegetables. Cook for another 5-7 minutes until chicken is cooked through and vegetables are tender.
5. Serve chicken and vegetables over brown rice.

Nutritional Information:

- Calories: 400; Fat: 10g; Protein: 30g; Carbs: 50g

Chapter 9 Lamb Recipes

Chapter 9 Lamb Recipes

Herb-Crusted Lamb Chops

Benefits: These Herb-Crusted Lamb Chops are packed with flavor and nutrients. The fresh herbs enhance the lamb's natural taste while providing antioxidants, making it a great choice for a healthy meal.

Servings: 4
Preparation Time: 15 minutes
Cooking Time: 20 minutes

Ingredients:

- 8 lamb chops, about 1-inch thick
- 2 tablespoons fresh rosemary, chopped
- 2 tablespoons fresh thyme, chopped
- 4 cloves garlic, minced
- 3 tablespoons olive oil
- Salt and pepper to taste

Instructions:

1. Preheat the oven to 400°F (200°C).
2. In a bowl, mix rosemary, thyme, garlic, olive oil, salt, and pepper to create a herb paste.
3. Rub the herb mixture generously over each lamb chop.
4. Heat an oven-safe skillet over medium-high heat. Add the lamb chops and sear for 3-4 minutes on each side until browned.
5. Transfer the skillet to the preheated oven and roast for 8-10 minutes for medium-rare.
6. Let the chops rest for 5 minutes before serving.

Nutritional Information:

- Calories: 320; Fat: 22g; Protein: 28g; Carbs: 2g

Moroccan Lamb Stew

Benefits: This Moroccan Lamb Stew is rich in flavor and nutrients, thanks to the combination of spices and vegetables. It's a comforting dish that's perfect for meal prep and keeps well in the fridge.

Servings: 6
Preparation Time: 20 minutes
Cooking Time: 2 hours

Ingredients:

- 2 pounds lamb shoulder, cubed
- 1 onion, diced
- 3 cloves garlic, minced
- 2 carrots, sliced
- 1 can (14 oz) chickpeas, drained
- 1 can (14 oz) diced tomatoes
- 2 cups low-sodium vegetable broth
- 1 tablespoon cumin
- 1 tablespoon coriander
- 1 teaspoon cinnamon
- Salt and pepper to taste
- 2 tablespoons olive oil
- Fresh cilantro, for garnish

Instructions:

1. In a large pot, heat olive oil over medium heat. Add onion and garlic; sauté until soft.
2. Add cubed lamb and brown on all sides.
3. Stir in carrots, chickpeas, diced tomatoes, vegetable broth, cumin, coriander, cinnamon, salt, and pepper.
4. Bring to a boil, then reduce heat to low. Cover and simmer for about 1.5 hours, stirring occasionally.
5. Once the lamb is tender, serve hot, garnished with fresh cilantro.

Nutritional Information:

- Calories: 450; Fat: 18g; Protein: 32g; Carbs: 36g

Spicy Lamb Meatballs

Benefits: These Spicy Lamb Meatballs are full of flavor and easy to make. The use of spices not only adds heat but also enhances metabolism, making this dish a great option for a protein-packed meal.

Servings: 4
Preparation Time: 15 minutes
Cooking Time: 25 minutes

Ingredients:

- 1 pound ground lamb
- 1/2 cup onion, finely chopped
- 2 cloves garlic, minced
- 1 teaspoon cumin
- 1 teaspoon paprika
- 1/2 teaspoon red pepper flakes
- 1/2 teaspoon salt
- 1/4 teaspoon black pepper
- 1/4 cup fresh parsley, chopped
- 2 tablespoons olive oil

Instructions:

1. Preheat the oven to 400°F (200°C).
2. In a bowl, combine ground lamb, onion, garlic, cumin, paprika, red pepper flakes, salt, black pepper, and parsley. Mix well.
3. Form the mixture into 1-inch meatballs and place them on a baking sheet.
4. Drizzle with olive oil and bake for 20-25 minutes, until browned and cooked through.
5. Serve with a side of fresh vegetables or over a bed of quinoa.

Nutritional Information:

- Calories: 300; Fat: 20g; Protein: 25g; Carbs: 5g

Grilled Lamb Kabobs

Benefits: These Grilled Lamb Kabobs are not only visually appealing but also packed with nutrients. Grilling helps retain the lamb's natural flavor while adding a smoky touch.

Servings: 4
Preparation Time: 30 minutes
Cooking Time: 15 minutes

Ingredients:

- 1.5 pounds lamb leg, cubed
- 1 bell pepper, chopped
- 1 red onion, chopped
- 1 zucchini, sliced
- 1/4 cup olive oil
- 2 tablespoons lemon juice
- 2 teaspoons garlic powder
- 1 teaspoon dried oregano
- Salt and pepper to taste
- Skewers (if using wooden, soak in water for 30 minutes)

Instructions:

1. In a bowl, whisk together olive oil, lemon juice, garlic powder, oregano, salt, and pepper.
2. Add the cubed lamb and vegetables to the marinade, tossing to coat. Allow to marinate for at least 30 minutes.
3. Preheat the grill to medium-high heat.
4. Thread lamb and vegetables onto skewers.
5. Grill kabobs for about 12-15 minutes, turning occasionally, until lamb is cooked to desired doneness.
6. Serve with a side of whole grains or a fresh salad.

Nutritional Information:

- Calories: 400; Fat: 25g; Protein: 30g; Carbs: 10g

Lamb and Sweet Potato Shepherd's Pie

Benefits: This Lamb and Sweet Potato Shepherd's Pie is a comforting, hearty dish that offers a healthy twist on a classic. Sweet potatoes provide vitamins and fiber, making this a nutrient-dense meal.

Servings: 6
Preparation Time: 20 minutes
Cooking Time: 40 minutes

Ingredients:

- 1 pound ground lamb
- 2 large sweet potatoes, peeled and cubed

- 1 cup carrots, diced
- 1 cup peas (fresh or frozen)
- 1 onion, diced
- 2 cloves garlic, minced
- 1 tablespoon tomato paste
- 1 cup low-sodium chicken broth
- 1 tablespoon olive oil
- Salt and pepper to taste

Instructions:

1. Preheat the oven to 375°F (190°C).
2. Boil sweet potatoes in a pot of salted water until tender, about 15 minutes. Drain and mash with a bit of olive oil, salt, and pepper. Set aside.
3. In a skillet, heat olive oil over medium heat. Add onion and garlic; sauté until soft.
4. Add ground lamb, carrots, tomato paste, chicken broth, salt, and pepper. Cook until lamb is browned and carrots are tender, about 10 minutes.
5. In a baking dish, layer the lamb mixture, then top with mashed sweet potatoes. Bake for 20 minutes until heated through.
6. Serve warm.

Nutritional Information:

- Calories: 420; Fat: 15g; Protein: 28g; Carbs: 45g

Lamb Tagine with Apricots

Benefits: This Lamb Tagine with Apricots combines savory and sweet flavors, providing a unique taste experience. The dried apricots add natural sweetness and are rich in vitamins and minerals.

Servings: 4
Preparation Time: 15 minutes
Cooking Time: 1.5 hours

Ingredients:

- 1.5 pounds lamb shanks
- 1 onion, chopped
- 2 cloves garlic, minced
- 1 teaspoon cumin
- 1 teaspoon cinnamon
- 1/2 teaspoon turmeric
- 1/2 cup dried apricots, chopped
- 2 cups low-sodium chicken broth
- 1 tablespoon olive oil
- Salt and pepper to taste
- Fresh cilantro for garnish

Instructions:

1. In a large pot, heat olive oil over medium heat. Add onion and garlic; sauté until soft.
2. Add lamb shanks and brown on all sides.
3. Stir in cumin, cinnamon, turmeric, salt, and pepper.
4. Add dried apricots and chicken broth; bring to a boil.
5. Reduce heat, cover, and simmer for about 1.5 hours, until the lamb is tender.
6. Serve with whole grains or vegetables, garnished with fresh cilantro.

Nutritional Information:

- Calories: 500; Fat: 25g; Protein: 45g; Carbs: 30g

Spiced Lamb and Quinoa Salad

Benefits: This Spiced Lamb and Quinoa Salad is a nutritious and filling meal, rich in protein and fiber. Quinoa adds a complete source of protein, making this dish great for energy and muscle recovery.

Servings: 4
Preparation Time: 15 minutes
Cooking Time: 20 minutes

Ingredients:

- 1 pound ground lamb
- 1 cup quinoa
- 2 cups water
- 1 cucumber, diced
- 1 cup cherry tomatoes, halved
- 1/4 cup red onion, diced
- 1 tablespoon cumin
- 1 tablespoon olive oil
- Salt and pepper to taste
- Fresh parsley for garnish

Instructions:

1. Rinse quinoa under cold water. In a saucepan, combine quinoa and water; bring to a boil. Reduce heat, cover, and simmer for 15 minutes until quinoa is fluffy.
2. In a skillet, heat olive oil over medium heat. Add ground lamb, cumin, salt, and pepper; cook until browned.
3. In a large bowl, combine cooked quinoa, cucumber, cherry tomatoes, red onion, and cooked lamb. Toss to mix.
4. Garnish with fresh parsley and serve warm or chilled.

Nutritional Information:

- Calories: 350; Fat: 18g; Protein: 25g; Carbs: 30g

Lamb and Spinach Stuffed Peppers

Benefits: These Lamb and Spinach Stuffed Peppers are a colorful, nutrient-rich meal. They provide a good balance of protein, fiber, and vitamins, making them perfect for a healthy diet.

Servings: 4
Preparation Time: 20 minutes
Cooking Time: 30 minutes

Ingredients:

- 4 bell peppers, halved and seeded
- 1 pound ground lamb
- 2 cups spinach, chopped
- 1 cup cooked brown rice
- 1 teaspoon garlic powder
- 1 teaspoon Italian seasoning
- Salt and pepper to taste
- 1 tablespoon olive oil
- 1/2 cup low-sodium tomato sauce

Instructions:

1. Preheat the oven to 375°F (190°C).
2. In a skillet, heat olive oil over medium heat. Add ground lamb and cook until browned.
3. Stir in chopped spinach, cooked rice, garlic powder, Italian seasoning, salt, and pepper. Cook for 2-3 minutes until spinach wilts.
4. Fill each bell pepper half with the lamb mixture and place in a baking dish.
5. Pour tomato sauce over the stuffed peppers and cover with foil. Bake for 25-30 minutes until peppers are tender.
6. Serve warm.

Nutritional Information:

- Calories: 280; Fat: 16g; Protein: 22g; Carbs: 20g

Lamb Curry with Coconut Milk

Benefits: This Lamb Curry with Coconut Milk is rich and creamy, offering a delightful blend of spices and flavors. Coconut milk provides healthy fats, making it a satisfying and hearty dish.

Servings: 4
Preparation Time: 15 minutes
Cooking Time: 40 minutes

Ingredients:

- 1.5 pounds lamb, cubed
- 1 onion, chopped
- 2 cloves garlic, minced
- 1 tablespoon ginger, grated
- 2 tablespoons curry powder
- 1 can (14 oz) coconut milk
- 2 cups low-sodium chicken broth
- 2 tablespoons olive oil
- Salt and pepper to taste
- Fresh cilantro for garnish

Instructions:

1. In a large pot, heat olive oil over medium heat. Add onion, garlic, and ginger; sauté until fragrant.
2. Add lamb cubes and brown on all sides.
3. Stir in curry powder, salt, and pepper.
4. Pour in coconut milk and chicken broth; bring to a boil.
5. Reduce heat and simmer for 30 minutes until lamb is tender.
6. Serve garnished with fresh cilantro, alongside whole grains or vegetables.

Nutritional Information:

- Calories: 500; Fat: 35g; Protein: 40g; Carbs: 10g

Lamb Burgers with Sweet Potato Fries

Benefits: These Lamb Burgers with Sweet Potato Fries provide a delicious and satisfying meal. Sweet potatoes offer complex carbohydrates and fiber, making this dish balanced and nutritious.

Servings: 4
Preparation Time: 20 minutes
Cooking Time: 30 minutes

Ingredients:

- 1 pound ground lamb
- 1/4 cup red onion, finely chopped
- 1 tablespoon fresh mint, chopped
- Salt and pepper to taste
- 2 large sweet potatoes, cut into fries
- 2 tablespoons olive oil

Instructions:

1. Preheat the oven to 425°F (220°C). Toss sweet potato fries in olive oil, salt, and pepper, then spread on a baking sheet. Bake for 25-30 minutes until crispy.
2. In a bowl, combine ground lamb, red onion, mint, salt, and pepper. Form into patties.
3. Cook lamb patties on a grill or skillet over medium heat for about 5-6 minutes on each side until cooked through.

4. Serve with baked sweet potato fries.

Nutritional Information:

- Calories: 450; Fat: 30g; Protein: 25g; Carbs: 35g

Lamb Tacos with Avocado Salsa

Benefits: These Lamb Tacos with Avocado Salsa are a fresh and healthy take on traditional tacos. Using lettuce as a wrap makes them lower in carbs, while avocado adds healthy fats and fiber.

Servings: 4
Preparation Time: 15 minutes
Cooking Time: 15 minutes

Ingredients:

- 1 pound ground lamb
- 1 tablespoon chili powder
- 1 teaspoon cumin
- Salt and pepper to taste
- 8 lettuce leaves (for wrapping)
- 1 avocado, diced
- 1 tomato, diced
- 1/4 red onion, chopped
- 1 lime, juiced

Instructions:

1. In a skillet over medium heat, cook ground lamb with chili powder, cumin, salt, and pepper until browned.
2. In a bowl, combine avocado, tomato, red onion, lime juice, and a pinch of salt to make the salsa.
3. Serve lamb in lettuce leaves, topped with avocado salsa.

Nutritional Information:

- Calories: 350; Fat: 25g; Protein: 25g; Carbs: 10g

Lamb and Vegetable Stir-Fry

Benefits: This Lamb and Vegetable Stir-Fry is a quick and nutritious meal packed with vitamins and minerals. The variety of vegetables enhances its health benefits, making it a great choice for busy days.

Servings: 4
Preparation Time: 15 minutes
Cooking Time: 15 minutes

Ingredients:

- 1 pound lamb, thinly sliced
- 2 cups mixed vegetables (bell peppers, broccoli, snap peas)
- 2 cloves garlic, minced
- 1 tablespoon ginger, minced
- 3 tablespoons low-sodium soy sauce
- 1 tablespoon sesame oil
- 1 tablespoon olive oil
- Salt and pepper to taste

Instructions:

1. In a wok or large skillet, heat olive oil over medium-high heat.
2. Add garlic and ginger; sauté for 1 minute until fragrant.
3. Add sliced lamb and cook until browned, about 5-7 minutes.
4. Stir in mixed vegetables and cook for another 5 minutes until tender-crisp.
5. Drizzle with soy sauce and sesame oil; stir well to combine. Serve hot.

Nutritional Information:

- Calories: 400; Fat: 25g; Protein: 30g; Carbs: 15g

Grilled Lamb Flatbreads

Benefits: These Grilled Lamb Flatbreads are a fun and interactive meal. The whole grains provide fiber, while the Greek yogurt adds protein and probiotics, promoting gut health.

Servings: 4
Preparation Time: 15 minutes
Cooking Time: 15 minutes

Ingredients:

- 1 pound ground lamb
- 1 tablespoon cumin
- 1 teaspoon paprika
- Salt and pepper to taste
- 4 whole grain flatbreads
- 1/2 cup Greek yogurt
- 1 cucumber, diced
- 1 cup cherry tomatoes, halved
- Fresh mint for garnish

Instructions:

1. In a skillet, cook ground lamb with cumin, paprika, salt, and pepper until browned.
2. Warm the flatbreads on a grill or skillet.
3. Spread a layer of Greek yogurt on each flatbread.
4. Top with cooked lamb, diced cucumber, and cherry tomatoes.
5. Garnish with fresh mint and serve warm.

Nutritional Information:

- Calories: 400; Fat: 20g; Protein: 30g; Carbs: 35g

Lamb and Lentil Soup

Benefits: This Lamb and Lentil Soup is hearty and packed with protein and fiber. Lentils are a great source of plant-based protein, making this soup nutritious and filling.

Servings: 6
Preparation Time: 15 minutes
Cooking Time: 45 minutes

Ingredients:

- 1 pound ground lamb
- 1 onion, chopped
- 2 cloves garlic, minced
- 2 carrots, diced
- 1 cup lentils (green or brown)
- 4 cups low-sodium vegetable broth
- 1 teaspoon thyme
- Salt and pepper to taste
- 1 tablespoon olive oil

Instructions:

1. In a large pot, heat olive oil over medium heat. Add onion and garlic; sauté until soft.
2. Add ground lamb and cook until browned.
3. Stir in carrots, lentils, broth, thyme, salt, and pepper.
4. Bring to a boil, then reduce heat and simmer for about 30 minutes, until lentils are tender.
5. Serve hot, garnished with fresh herbs if desired.

Nutritional Information:

- Calories: 350; Fat: 15g; Protein: 30g; Carbs: 30g

Lamb Bolognese with Zucchini Noodles

Benefits: This Lamb Bolognese with Zucchini Noodles is a healthier take on a classic dish. Using zucchini noodles cuts down on carbs while providing extra vegetables, making this a low-calorie yet satisfying meal.

Servings: 4
Preparation Time: 15 minutes
Cooking Time: 30 minutes

Ingredients:

- 1 pound ground lamb
- 1 onion, chopped
- 2 cloves garlic, minced
- 2 cups crushed tomatoes
- 1 teaspoon oregano
- 4 large zucchinis, spiralized
- Salt and pepper to taste
- 2 tablespoons olive oil

Instructions:

1. In a skillet, heat olive oil over medium heat. Add onion and garlic; sauté until softened.
2. Add ground lamb and cook until browned.
3. Stir in crushed tomatoes, oregano, salt, and pepper. Simmer for 20 minutes.
4. In a separate pan, lightly sauté spiralized zucchini for 2-3 minutes until tender.
5. Serve the lamb Bolognese over zucchini noodles.

Nutritional Information:

- Calories: 350; Fat: 20g; Protein: 30g; Carbs: 15g

Chapter 10 Pork Recipes

Chapter 10 Pork Recipes

Herb-Roasted Pork Tenderloin

Benefits: This Herb-Roasted Pork Tenderloin is rich in protein and low in carbs, making it an excellent choice for muscle maintenance and energy. The fresh herbs enhance flavor without added calories or unhealthy ingredients.

Servings: 4
Preparation Time: 15 minutes
Cooking Time: 25 minutes

Ingredients:

- 1 pound pork tenderloin
- 2 tablespoons olive oil
- 2 tablespoons fresh rosemary, chopped
- 2 tablespoons fresh thyme, chopped
- 4 cloves garlic, minced
- Salt and pepper to taste
- 1 lemon, zested and juiced

Instructions:

1. Preheat the oven to 400°F (200°C).
2. In a small bowl, mix olive oil, rosemary, thyme, garlic, lemon zest, salt, and pepper.
3. Rub the mixture over the pork tenderloin.
4. Place the tenderloin in a baking dish and roast for 20-25 minutes until the internal temperature reaches 145°F (63°C).
5. Let rest for 5 minutes before slicing. Serve with lemon juice drizzled on top.

Nutritional Information:

- Calories: 320; Fat: 15g; Protein: 40g; Carbs: 2g

Thai Pork and Vegetable Stir-Fry

Benefits: This Thai Pork and Vegetable Stir-Fry is packed with colorful veggies, providing essential vitamins and minerals. The coconut aminos offer a savory depth without the sodium found in traditional soy sauce, making this dish heart-healthy.

Servings: 4
Preparation Time: 15 minutes
Cooking Time: 10 minutes

Ingredients:

- 1 pound pork loin, thinly sliced
- 2 cups mixed vegetables (bell peppers, broccoli, carrots)
- 2 tablespoons coconut aminos
- 1 tablespoon ginger, minced
- 2 cloves garlic, minced
- 1 tablespoon olive oil
- Salt and pepper to taste
- Fresh cilantro for garnish

Instructions:

1. Heat olive oil in a large skillet or wok over medium-high heat.
2. Add ginger and garlic; sauté for 1 minute until fragrant.
3. Add sliced pork and cook until browned, about 3-4 minutes.
4. Stir in mixed vegetables and coconut aminos; cook for another 5 minutes until vegetables are tender.
5. Serve hot, garnished with fresh cilantro.

Nutritional Information:

- Calories: 380; Fat: 15g; Protein: 35g; Carbs: 25g

Garlic-Infused Pork Chops with Sweet Potato Mash

Benefits: Garlic-Infused Pork Chops with Sweet Potato Mash are a comforting yet nutritious meal. Sweet potatoes provide fiber and essential nutrients, while garlic is known for its immune-boosting properties.

Servings: 4
Preparation Time: 10 minutes
Cooking Time: 25 minutes

Ingredients:

- 4 bone-in pork chops
- 4 cloves garlic, minced
- 2 tablespoons olive oil
- Salt and pepper to taste
- 2 large sweet potatoes, peeled and cubed
- 1/4 cup almond milk (unsweetened)
- 1 teaspoon cinnamon

Instructions:

1. Preheat the oven to 375°F (190°C).
2. Season pork chops with salt, pepper, and minced garlic.
3. In a skillet, heat olive oil over medium-high heat. Sear pork chops for 3-4 minutes on each side until golden brown.
4. Transfer to the oven and bake for 15 minutes until cooked through.
5. Meanwhile, boil sweet potatoes until tender, about 15 minutes. Drain and mash with almond milk and cinnamon.
6. Serve pork chops with sweet potato mash.

Nutritional Information:

- Calories: 450; Fat: 25g; Protein: 30g; Carbs: 35g

Maple-Glazed Pork Belly with Roasted Brussels Sprouts

Benefits: Maple-Glazed Pork Belly with Roasted Brussels Sprouts is a flavorful dish that satisfies the palate. Brussels sprouts provide fiber and antioxidants, while the maple glaze offers natural sweetness without refined sugars.

Servings: 4
Preparation Time: 15 minutes
Cooking Time: 40 minutes

Ingredients:

- 1 pound pork belly, sliced
- 1/4 cup pure maple syrup
- 2 tablespoons soy sauce (low sodium)
- 1 teaspoon garlic powder
- 1 pound Brussels sprouts, halved
- 2 tablespoons olive oil
- Salt and pepper to taste

Instructions:

1. Preheat the oven to 400°F (200°C).
2. In a bowl, mix maple syrup, soy sauce, garlic powder, salt, and pepper.
3. Place pork belly slices in a baking dish and pour the glaze over them.
4. Toss Brussels sprouts with olive oil, salt, and pepper; place around the pork belly.
5. Bake for 30-35 minutes until pork is crispy and Brussels sprouts are tender.

Nutritional Information:

- Calories: 550; Fat: 40g; Protein: 25g; Carbs: 30g

Pork and Cauliflower Rice Stir-Fry

Benefits: This Pork and Cauliflower Rice Stir-Fry is a low-carb alternative to traditional fried rice. Cauliflower rice is a great way to increase vegetable intake while keeping the dish light and healthy.

Servings: 4
Preparation Time: 15 minutes
Cooking Time: 10 minutes

Ingredients:

- 1 pound pork tenderloin, diced
- 4 cups cauliflower rice
- 2 tablespoons olive oil
- 1 tablespoon ginger, minced
- 2 cloves garlic, minced
- 1/4 cup green onions, sliced
- Salt and pepper to taste

Instructions:

1. Heat olive oil in a large skillet over medium heat.
2. Add ginger and garlic; sauté for 1 minute.
3. Add diced pork and cook until browned.
4. Stir in cauliflower rice, salt, and pepper; cook for another 5-7 minutes until cauliflower is tender.
5. Garnish with green onions before serving.

Nutritional Information:

- Calories: 380; Fat: 20g; Protein: 30g; Carbs: 15g

Balsamic Glazed Pork Medallions

Benefits: Balsamic Glazed Pork Medallions are a quick and elegant dish that's full of flavor. Balsamic vinegar adds a rich taste without unhealthy additives, making it perfect for a light dinner.

Servings: 4
Preparation Time: 10 minutes
Cooking Time: 15 minutes

Ingredients:

- 1 pound pork tenderloin, sliced into medallions
- 1/4 cup balsamic vinegar
- 2 tablespoons honey (or maple syrup)
- 1 tablespoon olive oil
- Salt and pepper to taste
- 1 teaspoon rosemary, chopped

Instructions:

1. In a small bowl, whisk together balsamic vinegar, honey, olive oil, rosemary, salt, and pepper.
2. Heat a skillet over medium heat. Add pork medallions and cook for 3-4 minutes on each side until browned.
3. Pour the balsamic mixture over the pork and cook for an additional 2 minutes until glazed.
4. Serve warm with steamed vegetables.

Nutritional Information:

- Calories: 320; Fat: 12g; Protein: 35g; Carbs: 15g

Mediterranean Stuffed Pork Tenderloin

Benefits: Mediterranean Stuffed Pork Tenderloin is a flavorful, protein-packed dish. The combination of spinach and feta provides antioxidants and healthy fats, promoting overall wellness.

Servings: 4
Preparation Time: 20 minutes
Cooking Time: 30 minutes

Ingredients:

- 1 pound pork tenderloin
- 1 cup spinach, chopped
- 1/2 cup feta cheese, crumbled
- 1/4 cup sun-dried tomatoes, chopped
- 2 tablespoons olive oil
- Salt and pepper to taste

Instructions:

1. Preheat the oven to 375°F (190°C).
2. Butterfly the pork tenderloin and flatten it.
3. In a bowl, mix spinach, feta, sun-dried tomatoes, salt, and pepper.
4. Spread the mixture on the pork and roll it up tightly. Secure with kitchen twine.
5. Heat olive oil in an oven-safe skillet; sear the rolled pork on all sides.
6. Transfer to the oven and bake for 20-25 minutes until cooked through.

Nutritional Information:

- Calories: 450; Fat: 25g; Protein: 40g; Carbs: 10g

Pork and Apple Skillet

Benefits: This Pork and Apple Skillet combines savory and sweet flavors, providing a nutritious meal with the goodness of fruits. Apples add fiber and vitamins, making it a balanced dish.

Servings: 4
Preparation Time: 10 minutes
Cooking Time: 20 minutes

Ingredients:

- 1 pound pork chops, cubed
- 2 apples, diced
- 1 onion, sliced
- 2 tablespoons olive oil
- 1 teaspoon cinnamon
- Salt and pepper to taste

Instructions:

- Heat olive oil in a skillet over medium heat.
- Add onion and sauté until translucent.
- Add cubed pork and cook until browned.
- Stir in diced apples, cinnamon, salt, and pepper; cook for an additional 10 minutes until apples are tender.
- Serve warm, garnished with fresh herbs if desired.

Nutritional Information:

- Calories: 400; Fat: 20g; Protein: 30g; Carbs: 30g

Pork and Quinoa Stuffed Bell Peppers

Benefits: Pork and Quinoa Stuffed Bell Peppers provide a balanced meal rich in protein and fiber. Quinoa is a complete protein source, and the peppers add a dose of vitamins and antioxidants.

Servings: 4
Preparation Time: 15 minutes
Cooking Time: 35 minutes

Ingredients:

- 1 pound ground pork
- 1 cup cooked quinoa
- 4 large bell peppers, halved and seeded
- 1 can diced tomatoes (no added sugar)
- 1 teaspoon cumin
- Salt and pepper to taste
- 1 tablespoon olive oil

Instructions:

1. Preheat the oven to 375°F (190°C).
2. In a skillet, heat olive oil and brown ground pork.
3. Add cooked quinoa, diced tomatoes, cumin, salt, and pepper; mix well.
4. Stuff bell pepper halves with the pork mixture.
5. Place in a baking dish and bake for 25-30 minutes until peppers are tender.

Nutritional Information:

- Calories: 380; Fat: 15g; Protein: 30g; Carbs: 35g

Pork Tacos with Cabbage Slaw

Benefits: These Pork Tacos with Cabbage Slaw are a fun and nutritious meal. The cabbage slaw adds crunch and is high in fiber, while the pork provides a hearty protein source.

Servings: 4
Preparation Time: 15 minutes
Cooking Time: 15 minutes

Ingredients:

- 1 pound pork shoulder, shredded
- 1 tablespoon chili powder
- 1 teaspoon cumin
- 1/4 cup apple cider vinegar
- 2 cups cabbage, shredded
- 1 carrot, grated
- 8 corn tortillas

Instructions:

1. In a slow cooker, combine shredded pork, chili powder, cumin, and apple cider vinegar. Cook on low for 6 hours or high for 3 hours.
2. In a bowl, mix cabbage and carrot for the slaw.
3. Warm corn tortillas in a skillet.
4. Assemble tacos with shredded pork and top with cabbage slaw.

Nutritional Information:

- Calories: 420; Fat: 20g; Protein: 30g; Carbs: 35g

Smoky Pork and Black Bean Chili

Benefits: Smoky Pork and Black Bean Chili is hearty and satisfying, packed with protein and fiber. The black beans provide a great source of plant-based protein and essential nutrients.

Servings: 6
Preparation Time: 15 minutes
Cooking Time: 45 minutes

Ingredients:

- 1 pound ground pork
- 1 can black beans, rinsed and drained
- 1 can diced tomatoes (no added sugar)
- 1 onion, chopped
- 2 cloves garlic, minced
- 2 tablespoons chili powder
- 1 teaspoon smoked paprika
- Salt and pepper to taste

Instructions:

1. In a large pot, cook ground pork over medium heat until browned.
2. Add onion and garlic; sauté until softened.
3. Stir in black beans, diced tomatoes, chili powder, smoked paprika, salt, and pepper.
4. Simmer for 30 minutes, stirring occasionally.
5. Serve warm with fresh cilantro.

Nutritional Information:

- Calories: 350; Fat: 15g; Protein: 30g; Carbs: 25g

Pork and Vegetable Sheet Pan Dinner

Benefits: This Pork and Vegetable Sheet Pan Dinner is a quick, easy, and nutritious meal. One-pan meals simplify cleanup and allow for a variety of colorful vegetables, boosting your nutrient intake.

Servings: 4
Preparation Time: 15 minutes
Cooking Time: 30 minutes

Ingredients:

- 1 pound pork chops
- 2 cups mixed vegetables (zucchini, bell peppers, carrots)
- 2 tablespoons olive oil
- 1 teaspoon garlic powder
- Salt and pepper to taste

Instructions:

1. Preheat the oven to 425°F (220°C).
2. On a sheet pan, arrange pork chops and mixed vegetables.
3. Drizzle with olive oil, sprinkle garlic powder, salt, and pepper.
4. Toss to coat, then spread evenly.
5. Roast for 25-30 minutes until the pork is cooked through and the vegetables are tender.

Nutritional Information:

- Calories: 400; Fat: 20g; Protein: 30g; Carbs: 20g

Pork and Spinach Frittata

Benefits: Pork and Spinach Frittata is a protein-packed breakfast or brunch option. It's easy to make, full of nutrients, and can be customized with various vegetables.

Servings: 4
Preparation Time: 10 minutes
Cooking Time: 25 minutes

Ingredients:

- 1 pound ground pork
- 6 eggs
- 2 cups spinach, chopped
- 1/4 cup almond milk (unsweetened)
- 1 teaspoon garlic powder
- Salt and pepper to taste
- 1 tablespoon olive oil

Instructions:

1. Preheat the oven to 350°F (175°C).
2. In an oven-safe skillet, heat olive oil and cook ground pork until browned.
3. Stir in spinach and cook until wilted.
4. In a bowl, whisk together eggs, almond milk, garlic powder, salt, and pepper.
5. Pour egg mixture over pork and spinach. Cook for 5 minutes, then transfer to the oven and bake for 15-20 minutes until set.

Nutritional Information:

- Calories: 350; Fat: 25g; Protein: 30g; Carbs: 5g

Spicy Pork Lettuce Wraps

Benefits: These Spicy Pork Lettuce Wraps are a fun and healthy alternative to traditional wraps. Using lettuce instead of tortillas reduces carbs and calories while keeping the meal fresh and satisfying.

Servings: 4
Preparation Time: 15 minutes
Cooking Time: 10 minutes

Ingredients:

- 1 pound ground pork
- 1 tablespoon chili powder
- 1 tablespoon cumin
- 1 tablespoon olive oil
- 1/4 cup green onions, chopped
- 1 tablespoon fresh cilantro, chopped
- 8 large lettuce leaves (for wrapping)
- Salt and pepper to taste

Instructions:

1. Heat olive oil in a skillet over medium heat. Add ground pork, chili powder, cumin, salt, and pepper; cook until browned.
2. Stir in green onions and cilantro, cooking for an additional 2 minutes.
3. Spoon the pork mixture into lettuce leaves and serve immediately.

Nutritional Information:

- Calories: 320; Fat: 20g; Protein: 25g; Carbs: 5g

Pork Stir-Fry with Broccoli and Carrots

Benefits: This Pork Stir-Fry with Broccoli and Carrots is a quick and nutritious meal. Packed with colorful vegetables, it's rich in vitamins and minerals while providing a good protein source from the pork.

Servings: 4
Preparation Time: 10 minutes
Cooking Time: 15 minutes

Ingredients:

- 1 pound pork loin, thinly sliced
- 2 cups broccoli florets
- 2 carrots, sliced
- 2 tablespoons coconut aminos
- 1 tablespoon ginger, minced
- 2 cloves garlic, minced
- 1 tablespoon olive oil
- Salt and pepper to taste

Instructions:

1. Heat olive oil in a large skillet over medium heat.
2. Add ginger and garlic; sauté for 1 minute until fragrant.
3. Add sliced pork and cook until browned, about 4 minutes.
4. Stir in broccoli, carrots, and coconut aminos; cook for another 5-7 minutes until vegetables are tender.
5. Serve hot, garnished with sesame seeds if desired.

Nutritional Information:

- Calories: 380; Fat: 15g; Protein: 35g; Carbs: 25g

Chapter 11 Fish and Seafood Recipes

Chapter 11 Fish and Seafood Recipes

Grilled Lemon Herb Shrimp Skewers

Benefits: Grilled Lemon Herb Shrimp Skewers are a light and flavorful dish that's packed with protein. Shrimp are low in calories and rich in nutrients, making this a perfect choice for a healthy meal. The fresh herbs and lemon juice add a refreshing twist, enhancing the dish's overall flavor without unhealthy ingredients.

Servings: 4
Preparation Time: 15 minutes
Cooking Time: 10 minutes

Ingredients:

- 1 pound large shrimp, peeled and deveined
- 3 tablespoons olive oil
- 2 tablespoons fresh lemon juice
- 2 cloves garlic, minced
- 1 tablespoon fresh parsley, chopped
- 1 tablespoon fresh basil, chopped
- Salt and pepper to taste
- Lemon wedges for serving

Instructions:

1. In a bowl, combine olive oil, lemon juice, garlic, parsley, basil, salt, and pepper.
2. Add shrimp to the marinade, coating well. Allow to marinate for 15 minutes.
3. Preheat the grill to medium-high heat.
4. Thread shrimp onto skewers, leaving space between each shrimp.
5. Grill for about 2-3 minutes per side or until shrimp are pink and opaque.
6. Serve with lemon wedges.

Nutritional Information:

- Calories: 250; Fat: 15g; Protein: 25g; Carbs: 2g

Spicy Baked Salmon with Quinoa

Benefits: This Spicy Baked Salmon with Quinoa is not only delicious but also packed with omega-3 fatty acids, which are essential for heart health. Quinoa provides a complete protein source and fiber, making this dish satisfying and nutritious.

Servings: 4
Preparation Time: 10 minutes
Cooking Time: 20 minutes

Ingredients:

- 4 salmon fillets
- 2 tablespoons olive oil
- 1 tablespoon chili powder
- 1 teaspoon paprika
- 1/2 teaspoon garlic powder
- Salt and pepper to taste
- 1 cup cooked quinoa
- 2 cups steamed broccoli

Instructions:

1. Preheat the oven to 400°F (200°C).
2. In a small bowl, mix olive oil, chili powder, paprika, garlic powder, salt, and pepper.
3. Place salmon fillets on a baking sheet and brush with the spice mixture.
4. Bake for 15-20 minutes or until the salmon is cooked through and flakes easily with a fork.
5. Serve with cooked quinoa and steamed broccoli on the side.

Nutritional Information:

- Calories: 450; Fat: 25g; Protein: 35g; Carbs: 30g

Coconut Curry Mussels

Benefits: Coconut Curry Mussels are a creamy and aromatic dish that combines the health benefits of seafood with the richness of coconut milk. Mussels are a lean protein source and provide essential minerals, making this dish a great choice for a healthy meal.

Servings: 4
Preparation Time: 10 minutes
Cooking Time: 15 minutes

Ingredients:

- 2 pounds mussels, cleaned and debearded
- 1 can (13.5 oz) coconut milk
- 2 tablespoons red curry paste
- 1 tablespoon olive oil
- 3 cloves garlic, minced
- 1 tablespoon ginger, minced
- 1 tablespoon lime juice
- Fresh cilantro for garnish

Instructions:

1. In a large pot, heat olive oil over medium heat. Add garlic and ginger; sauté for 1-2 minutes until fragrant.
2. Stir in the red curry paste and cook for another minute.
3. Pour in the coconut milk and bring to a simmer.
4. Add mussels, cover the pot, and cook for 5-7 minutes until mussels open.
5. Remove from heat, stir in lime juice, and garnish with cilantro.

Nutritional Information:

- Calories: 300; Fat: 20g; Protein: 25g; Carbs: 10g

Garlic Butter Scallops with Zucchini Noodles

Benefits: Garlic Butter Scallops with Zucchini Noodles is a gourmet dish that is quick to prepare and incredibly satisfying. Zucchini noodles offer a low-carb alternative to pasta, making this meal light yet flavorful.

Servings: 4
Preparation Time: 10 minutes
Cooking Time: 10 minutes

Ingredients:

- 1 pound scallops
- 3 tablespoons grass-fed butter
- 4 cloves garlic, minced
- 2 medium zucchinis, spiralized
- Salt and pepper to taste

- Fresh parsley for garnish

Instructions:

1. In a skillet, melt butter over medium heat.
2. Add garlic and sauté for 1 minute until fragrant.
3. Season scallops with salt and pepper; add to the skillet and sear for 2-3 minutes per side until golden brown.
4. Add zucchini noodles to the skillet and toss for 2-3 minutes until just tender.
5. Serve scallops over zucchini noodles, garnished with parsley.

Nutritional Information:

- Calories: 320; Fat: 25g; Protein: 30g; Carbs: 10g

Lemon Garlic Tilapia with Asparagus

Benefits: Lemon Garlic Tilapia with Asparagus is a light and refreshing dish rich in protein and healthy fats. Tilapia is a lean fish that cooks quickly, and asparagus adds essential nutrients, making it an excellent choice for a healthy meal.

Servings: 4
Preparation Time: 10 minutes
Cooking Time: 15 minutes

Ingredients:

- 4 tilapia fillets
- 3 tablespoons olive oil
- 2 tablespoons lemon juice
- 3 cloves garlic, minced
- 1 pound asparagus, trimmed
- Salt and pepper to taste

Instructions:

1. Preheat the oven to 375°F (190°C).
2. In a small bowl, mix olive oil, lemon juice, garlic, salt, and pepper.
3. Place tilapia fillets and asparagus on a baking sheet; drizzle with the olive oil mixture.
4. Bake for 12-15 minutes or until tilapia is cooked through and asparagus is tender.
5. Serve immediately.

Nutritional Information:

- Calories: 280; Fat: 15g; Protein: 30g; Carbs: 10g

Shrimp and Avocado Salad

Benefits: Shrimp and Avocado Salad is a refreshing and nutrient-dense dish that's perfect for a light lunch or dinner. Avocados provide healthy fats and fiber, while shrimp adds a lean protein boost.

Servings: 4
Preparation Time: 15 minutes
Cooking Time: 0 minutes

Ingredients:

- 1 pound cooked shrimp, peeled and deveined
- 2 ripe avocados, diced
- 1 cup cherry tomatoes, halved
- 1/4 cup red onion, finely chopped
- 1/4 cup fresh cilantro, chopped
- 2 tablespoons lime juice
- Salt and pepper to taste

Instructions:

1. In a large bowl, combine shrimp, avocados, cherry tomatoes, red onion, and cilantro.
2. Drizzle with lime juice, then season with salt and pepper.
3. Gently toss to combine.
4. Serve chilled or at room temperature.

Nutritional Information:

- Calories: 350; Fat: 25g; Protein: 20g; Carbs: 15g

Teriyaki Glazed Salmon with Broccoli

Benefits: Teriyaki Glazed Salmon with Broccoli is a delightful meal that combines the rich flavors of salmon with the health benefits of vegetables. The coconut aminos offer a low-sodium alternative to soy sauce, keeping this dish heart-healthy.

Servings: 4
Preparation Time: 10 minutes
Cooking Time: 15 minutes

Ingredients:

- 4 salmon fillets
- 1/4 cup coconut aminos
- 2 tablespoons honey (or maple syrup)
- 1 tablespoon ginger, minced
- 2 cups broccoli florets
- 1 tablespoon sesame seeds for garnish

Instructions:

1. In a small bowl, mix coconut aminos, honey, and ginger to make the teriyaki glaze.
2. Preheat the oven to 400°F (200°C).
3. Place salmon fillets on a baking sheet and brush with the glaze.
4. Bake for 12-15 minutes until the salmon is cooked through.
5. Steam broccoli while the salmon cooks.
6. Serve salmon with broccoli, garnished with sesame seeds.

Nutritional Information:

- Calories: 400; Fat: 20g; Protein: 35g; Carbs: 15g

Shrimp and Vegetable Stir-Fry

Benefits: Shrimp and Vegetable Stir-Fry is a quick and nutritious meal that's perfect for busy weeknights. Packed with protein and colorful vegetables, it provides essential vitamins and minerals in every bite.

Servings: 4
Preparation Time: 10 minutes
Cooking Time: 10 minutes

Ingredients:

- 1 pound shrimp, peeled and deveined
- 2 cups mixed vegetables (bell peppers, snap peas, carrots)
- 2 tablespoons olive oil
- 2 tablespoons coconut aminos
- 2 cloves garlic, minced
- 1 teaspoon ginger, minced
- Salt and pepper to taste

Instructions:

1. Heat olive oil in a large skillet over medium heat.
2. Add garlic and ginger; sauté for 1 minute.
3. Add shrimp and cook until pink, about 3-4 minutes.
4. Add mixed vegetables and coconut aminos; stir-fry for an additional 2-3 minutes until vegetables are tender.
5. Season with salt and pepper, then serve hot.

Nutritional Information:

- Calories: 300; Fat: 15g; Protein: 30g; Carbs: 15g

Pesto Zoodles with Shrimp

Benefits: Pesto Zoodles with Shrimp is a flavorful and low-carb meal that's packed with nutrients. The homemade pesto adds healthy fats from nuts and olive oil, while zucchini noodles provide a fresh and light base.

Servings: 4
Preparation Time: 15 minutes
Cooking Time: 10 minutes

Ingredients:

- 1 pound shrimp, peeled and deveined
- 4 medium zucchinis, spiralized
- 1/2 cup homemade basil pesto (or store-bought without additives)
- 2 tablespoons olive oil
- Salt and pepper to taste
- Cherry tomatoes for garnish

Instructions:

1. In a skillet, heat olive oil over medium heat.
2. Add shrimp and cook until pink, about 3-4 minutes.
3. Remove shrimp from the skillet and set aside.
4. Add spiralized zucchini to the skillet; sauté for 2-3 minutes until tender.
5. Stir in pesto and cooked shrimp; mix until well combined.
6. Serve garnished with cherry tomatoes.

Nutritional Information:

- Calories: 350; Fat: 20g; Protein: 30g; Carbs: 15g

Shrimp and Cauliflower Rice Bowl

Benefits: Shrimp and Cauliflower Rice Bowl is a nutritious and satisfying meal that's low in carbs but high in flavor. Cauliflower rice is a great alternative to grains, providing fiber and essential nutrients without the extra calories.

Servings: 4
Preparation Time: 15 minutes
Cooking Time: 15 minutes

Ingredients:

- 1 pound shrimp, peeled and deveined
- 1 medium head cauliflower, grated into rice-sized pieces
- 1 cup bell peppers, diced
- 2 tablespoons olive oil
- 2 cloves garlic, minced
- Salt and pepper to taste
- Fresh cilantro for garnish

Instructions:

1. In a skillet, heat olive oil over medium heat.
2. Add garlic and sauté for 1 minute.
3. Add shrimp and cook until pink, about 3-4 minutes.
4. Remove shrimp and set aside.
5. Add cauliflower rice and bell peppers; sauté for 5-7 minutes until tender.
6. Stir in shrimp, season with salt and pepper, and garnish with cilantro before serving.

Nutritional Information:

- Calories: 280; Fat: 15g; Protein: 30g; Carbs: 10g

Miso Glazed Cod

Benefits: Miso Glazed Cod is a flavorful and healthy dish that's rich in omega-3 fatty acids and probiotics. The glaze adds depth of flavor while keeping the dish light and nutritious.

Servings: 4
Preparation Time: 10 minutes
Cooking Time: 15 minutes

Ingredients:

- 4 cod fillets
- 1/4 cup miso paste (white or yellow)
- 2 tablespoons maple syrup (or honey)
- 2 tablespoons rice vinegar
- 1 tablespoon sesame oil
- 1 teaspoon grated ginger

Instructions:

1. In a bowl, whisk together miso paste, maple syrup, rice vinegar, sesame oil, and ginger.
2. Preheat the oven to 400°F (200°C).
3. Place cod fillets on a baking sheet and brush generously with the miso glaze.
4. Bake for 12-15 minutes until fish is cooked through and flakes easily.
5. Serve hot, garnished with sesame seeds if desired.

Nutritional Information:

- Calories: 350; Fat: 15g; Protein: 35g; Carbs: 15g

Shrimp Tacos with Mango Salsa

Benefits: Shrimp Tacos with Mango Salsa are a fun and flavorful meal perfect for any occasion. The sweet mango salsa adds a refreshing contrast to the savory shrimp, making it a well-rounded dish that's both delicious and healthy.

Servings: 4
Preparation Time: 15 minutes
Cooking Time: 10 minutes

Ingredients:

- 1 pound shrimp, peeled and deveined
- 8 corn tortillas
- 1 cup diced mango
- 1/4 cup red onion, diced
- 1/4 cup cilantro, chopped
- 2 tablespoons lime juice
- Salt and pepper to taste

Instructions:

1. In a bowl, combine mango, red onion, cilantro, lime juice, salt, and pepper to make the salsa.
2. In a skillet, cook shrimp over medium heat until pink, about 3-4 minutes.
3. Warm corn tortillas in a separate skillet.
4. Assemble tacos with shrimp and top with mango salsa.

Nutritional Information:

- Calories: 320; Fat: 10g; Protein: 30g; Carbs: 30g

Grilled Fish Tacos with Cabbage Slaw

Benefits: Grilled Fish Tacos with Cabbage Slaw are a flavorful and healthy option for taco night. The fish provides lean protein, while the cabbage slaw adds crunch and essential nutrients without the extra calories.

Servings: 4
Preparation Time: 15 minutes
Cooking Time: 10 minutes

Ingredients:

- 1 pound white fish (like tilapia or cod)
- 1 tablespoon olive oil
- 1 tablespoon lime juice
- 1 teaspoon cumin
- 1/2 teaspoon paprika
- 8 corn tortillas
- 2 cups shredded cabbage
- 1/4 cup cilantro, chopped
- Salt and pepper to taste

Instructions:

1. Preheat the grill to medium heat.
2. In a bowl, mix olive oil, lime juice, cumin, paprika, salt, and pepper.
3. Brush the fish with the marinade and grill for 3-4 minutes per side until cooked through.
4. In another bowl, combine cabbage and cilantro.
5. Assemble tacos with grilled fish and top with cabbage slaw.

Nutritional Information:

- Calories: 320; Fat: 10g; Protein: 30g; Carbs: 25g

Clam Chowder with Cauliflower

Benefits: Clam Chowder with Cauliflower is a creamy and satisfying soup that's lower in carbs than traditional chowder. The cauliflower provides a nutrient-rich base, while clams are an excellent source of protein and minerals.

Servings: 4
Preparation Time: 10 minutes
Cooking Time: 30 minutes

Ingredients:

- 2 cans (6.5 oz each) chopped clams in juice
- 1 head cauliflower, chopped
- 1 onion, diced
- 2 cloves garlic, minced
- 2 cups vegetable broth
- 1 cup unsweetened almond milk
- 2 tablespoons olive oil
- Salt and pepper to taste

Instructions:

1. In a pot, heat olive oil over medium heat. Add onion and garlic; sauté until translucent.
2. Add cauliflower and vegetable broth; bring to a boil.
3. Reduce heat and simmer until cauliflower is tender, about 15 minutes.
4. Blend the soup until smooth; stir in almond milk and clams.
5. Season with salt and pepper before serving.

Nutritional Information:

- Calories: 250; Fat: 15g; Protein: 20g; Carbs: 15g

Honey Garlic Shrimp with Brown Rice

Benefits: Honey Garlic Shrimp with Brown Rice is a quick and satisfying meal that's perfect for weeknights. The dish combines sweet and savory flavors while providing essential nutrients, thanks to the shrimp and whole grains.

Servings: 4
Preparation Time: 10 minutes
Cooking Time: 15 minutes

Ingredients:

- 1 pound shrimp, peeled and deveined
- 2 tablespoons honey (or maple syrup)
- 3 cloves garlic, minced
- 2 tablespoons olive oil
- 2 cups cooked brown rice
- Salt and pepper to taste
- Green onions for garnish

Instructions:

1. In a bowl, mix honey, garlic, olive oil, salt, and pepper.
2. Heat a skillet over medium heat and add shrimp.
3. Pour the honey garlic mixture over shrimp and cook for 3-4 minutes until shrimp are pink.
4. Serve over cooked brown rice and garnish with green onions.

Nutritional Information:

- Calories: 400; Fat: 15g; Protein: 30g; Carbs: 40g

Chapter 12 Vegetarian Recipes

Chapter 12 Vegetarian Recipes

Quinoa and Black Bean Salad

Benefits: Quinoa and Black Bean Salad is a nutrient-dense dish packed with protein and fiber. Quinoa provides a complete protein source, while black beans add heartiness and essential nutrients. This salad is refreshing and perfect for meal prep.

Servings: 4
Preparation Time: 15 minutes
Cooking Time: 15 minutes

Ingredients:

- 1 cup quinoa, rinsed
- 2 cups water
- 1 can (15 oz) black beans, rinsed and drained
- 1 cup cherry tomatoes, halved
- 1 bell pepper, diced
- 1/4 cup red onion, finely chopped
- 1/4 cup fresh cilantro, chopped
- 1/4 cup lime juice
- 2 tablespoons olive oil
- Salt and pepper to taste

Instructions:

1. In a medium saucepan, combine quinoa and water. Bring to a boil, then reduce heat to low, cover, and simmer for about 15 minutes until quinoa is fluffy and water is absorbed.
2. In a large bowl, combine cooked quinoa, black beans, cherry tomatoes, bell pepper, red onion, and cilantro.
3. In a small bowl, whisk together lime juice, olive oil, salt, and pepper.
4. Pour the dressing over the salad and toss to combine. Serve chilled or at room temperature.

Nutritional Information:

- Calories: 350; Fat: 10g; Protein: 15g; Carbs: 55g

Sweet Potato and Chickpea Curry

Benefits: Sweet Potato and Chickpea Curry is a hearty and warming dish rich in vitamins and minerals. Sweet potatoes provide a natural sweetness and are high in beta-carotene, while chickpeas add protein and fiber, making this meal both satisfying and nutritious.

Servings: 4
Preparation Time: 10 minutes
Cooking Time: 30 minutes

Ingredients:

- 2 medium sweet potatoes, peeled and cubed
- 1 can (15 oz) chickpeas, rinsed and drained
- 1 onion, diced
- 2 cloves garlic, minced
- 1 tablespoon ginger, minced
- 1 can (14 oz) coconut milk
- 2 tablespoons curry powder
- 1 tablespoon olive oil
- Salt and pepper to taste
- Fresh cilantro for garnish

Instructions:

1. In a large pot, heat olive oil over medium heat. Add onion, garlic, and ginger; sauté until onion is translucent.
2. Stir in curry powder and cook for an additional minute.
3. Add sweet potatoes and chickpeas to the pot, stirring to coat.
4. Pour in coconut milk and bring to a boil. Reduce heat, cover, and simmer for about 20 minutes until sweet potatoes are tender.
5. Season with salt and pepper and garnish with fresh cilantro before serving.

Nutritional Information:

- Calories: 400; Fat: 18g; Protein: 12g; Carbs: 60g

Cauliflower Rice Stir-Fry

Benefits: Cauliflower Rice Stir-Fry is a low-carb alternative to traditional fried rice. Cauliflower is high in vitamins and minerals while providing a great base for stir-frying. This dish is quick to make and packed with colorful vegetables.

Servings: 4
Preparation Time: 10 minutes
Cooking Time: 10 minutes

Ingredients:

- 1 head cauliflower, grated into rice-sized pieces
- 1 cup mixed bell peppers, diced
- 1 cup broccoli florets
- 2 carrots, shredded
- 3 tablespoons coconut aminos
- 2 tablespoons sesame oil
- 2 cloves garlic, minced
- 1 teaspoon ginger, minced
- Salt and pepper to taste

Instructions:

1. In a large skillet or wok, heat sesame oil over medium heat.
2. Add garlic and ginger; sauté for 1 minute.
3. Add bell peppers, broccoli, and carrots; stir-fry for about 3-4 minutes until vegetables are tender.
4. Stir in cauliflower rice and coconut aminos; cook for another 5 minutes, stirring frequently.
5. Season with salt and pepper before serving.

Nutritional Information:

- Calories: 220; Fat: 12g; Protein: 6g; Carbs: 25g

Spinach and Mushroom Quiche

Benefits: Spinach and Mushroom Quiche is a nutritious and filling meal that can be enjoyed for breakfast, lunch, or dinner. Spinach provides iron and antioxidants, while mushrooms add depth of flavor and texture.

Servings: 6
Preparation Time: 15 minutes
Cooking Time: 35 minutes

Ingredients:

- 1 pre-made whole-grain pie crust
- 2 cups fresh spinach, chopped
- 1 cup mushrooms, sliced
- 4 eggs
- 1 cup unsweetened almond milk
- 1/2 teaspoon nutmeg
- Salt and pepper to taste
- 1/2 cup feta cheese (optional)

Instructions:

1. Preheat the oven to 375°F (190°C).
2. In a skillet, sauté mushrooms until soft, then add spinach and cook until wilted.
3. In a bowl, whisk together eggs, almond milk, nutmeg, salt, and pepper.
4. Spread the sautéed vegetables in the pie crust and pour the egg mixture over the top. Sprinkle with feta cheese if using.
5. Bake for 30-35 minutes, or until the quiche is set and golden. Let cool slightly before slicing.

Nutritional Information:

- Calories: 280; Fat: 18g; Protein: 12g; Carbs: 22g

Zucchini Noodles with Avocado Sauce

Benefits: Zucchini Noodles with Avocado Sauce is a creamy, low-carb alternative to traditional pasta. The avocado provides healthy fats and a rich, satisfying flavor, while zucchini adds fiber and essential vitamins.

Servings: 4
Preparation Time: 10 minutes
Cooking Time: 5 minutes

Ingredients:

- 4 medium zucchinis, spiralized
- 2 ripe avocados
- 1/4 cup fresh basil leaves
- 2 tablespoons lemon juice
- 2 cloves garlic, minced
- Salt and pepper to taste
- Cherry tomatoes for garnish

Instructions:

1. In a food processor, combine avocados, basil, lemon juice, garlic, salt, and pepper; blend until smooth.
2. In a skillet, lightly sauté zucchini noodles over medium heat for 2-3 minutes until just tender.
3. Remove from heat and toss with avocado sauce.
4. Serve immediately, garnished with cherry tomatoes.

Nutritional Information:

- Calories: 300; Fat: 22g; Protein: 6g; Carbs: 20g

Lentil and Vegetable Stew

Benefits: Lentil and Vegetable Stew is a hearty and warming dish that's perfect for any season. Lentils are an excellent source of plant-based protein and fiber, while the vegetables add essential nutrients and flavors.

Servings: 4
Preparation Time: 10 minutes
Cooking Time: 30 minutes

Ingredients:

- 1 cup lentils, rinsed
- 1 onion, diced
- 2 carrots, diced
- 2 celery stalks, diced
- 2 cloves garlic, minced
- 4 cups vegetable broth
- 1 can (14 oz) diced tomatoes
- 1 teaspoon thyme
- Salt and pepper to taste
- 2 tablespoons olive oil

Instructions:

1. In a large pot, heat olive oil over medium heat. Add onion, garlic, carrots, and celery; sauté until vegetables are softened.
2. Stir in lentils, diced tomatoes, vegetable broth, thyme, salt, and pepper.
3. Bring to a boil, then reduce heat and simmer for 25-30 minutes until lentils are tender.
4. Adjust seasoning before serving.

Nutritional Information:

- Calories: 350; Fat: 8g; Protein: 18g; Carbs: 60g

Roasted Vegetable Medley

Benefits: Roasted Vegetable Medley is a simple yet flavorful dish that showcases seasonal produce. Roasting enhances the natural sweetness of vegetables, making them a delicious side or a filling main course when served over whole grains.

Servings: 4
Preparation Time: 10 minutes
Cooking Time: 25 minutes

Ingredients:

- 1 cup Brussels sprouts, halved
- 1 cup carrots, sliced
- 1 cup bell peppers, diced
- 1 cup zucchini, diced
- 3 tablespoons olive oil
- 2 teaspoons dried herbs (like thyme or rosemary)
- Salt and pepper to taste

Instructions:

1. Preheat the oven to 425°F (220°C).
2. In a large bowl, toss all vegetables with olive oil, dried herbs, salt, and pepper.
3. Spread the vegetables on a baking sheet in a single layer.
4. Roast for 20-25 minutes, stirring halfway through, until vegetables are tender and slightly caramelized.
5. Serve warm as a side dish or over grains for a main dish.

Nutritional Information:

- Calories: 250; Fat: 15g; Protein: 5g; Carbs: 30g

Chickpea and Spinach Stew

Benefits: Chickpea and Spinach Stew is a protein-packed dish that's hearty and nutritious. Chickpeas provide fiber and protein, while spinach adds iron and vitamins, making it a balanced meal.

Servings: 4
Preparation Time: 10 minutes
Cooking Time: 20 minutes

Ingredients:

- 1 can (15 oz) chickpeas, rinsed and drained
- 2 cups fresh spinach, chopped
- 1 onion, diced
- 2 cloves garlic, minced
- 1 can (14 oz) diced tomatoes
- 1 teaspoon cumin
- 1 tablespoon olive oil
- Salt and pepper to taste

Instructions:

1. In a pot, heat olive oil over medium heat. Add onion and garlic, sautéing until the onion is translucent.
2. Stir in cumin, chickpeas, diced tomatoes, and salt. Simmer for about 10 minutes.
3. Add fresh spinach and cook until wilted. Adjust seasoning before serving.

Nutritional Information:

- Calories: 280; Fat: 8g; Protein: 15g; Carbs: 40g

Grilled Vegetable Skewers

Benefits: Grilled Vegetable Skewers are a colorful and flavorful addition to any meal. Grilling enhances the natural flavors of the vegetables, and they can be served as a side or added to salads or grain bowls.

Servings: 4
Preparation Time: 15 minutes
Cooking Time: 15 minutes

Ingredients:

- 1 zucchini, sliced
- 1 bell pepper, cubed
- 1 red onion, cubed
- 1 cup cherry tomatoes
- 2 tablespoons balsamic vinegar
- 2 tablespoons olive oil
- Salt and pepper to taste

Instructions:

1. Preheat the grill to medium-high heat.
2. In a large bowl, combine vegetables, balsamic vinegar, olive oil, salt, and pepper. Toss to coat.
3. Thread vegetables onto skewers.
4. Grill skewers for 10-15 minutes, turning occasionally until vegetables are tender and slightly charred.

Nutritional Information:

- Calories: 150; Fat: 8g; Protein: 3g; Carbs: 15g

Mediterranean Stuffed Peppers

Benefits: Mediterranean Stuffed Peppers are a vibrant and satisfying dish that's rich in flavors. The combination of brown rice, olives, and tomatoes provides a wealth of nutrients, making this a wholesome meal.

Servings: 4
Preparation Time: 15 minutes
Cooking Time: 30 minutes

Ingredients:

- 4 bell peppers, halved and seeds removed
- 1 cup cooked brown rice
- 1 can (15 oz) black olives, sliced
- 1 cup cherry tomatoes, halved
- 1 teaspoon oregano
- 1 tablespoon olive oil
- Salt and pepper to taste
- 1/2 cup feta cheese (optional)

Instructions:

1. Preheat the oven to 375°F (190°C).
2. In a bowl, mix cooked rice, olives, tomatoes, oregano, olive oil, salt, and pepper.
3. Stuff the bell pepper halves with the mixture.
4. Place in a baking dish and cover with foil. Bake for 25-30 minutes.
5. Remove foil, sprinkle with feta cheese if using, and bake for an additional 5 minutes until cheese is melted.

Nutritional Information:

- Calories: 320; Fat: 14g; Protein: 9g; Carbs: 45g

Beet and Goat Cheese Salad

Benefits: Beet and Goat Cheese Salad is a colorful dish full of antioxidants. Beets are known for their health benefits, including improved blood flow and lower blood pressure, while goat cheese adds creaminess and flavor.

Servings: 4
Preparation Time: 10 minutes
Cooking Time: 30 minutes

Ingredients:

- 4 medium beets, roasted and sliced
- 4 cups mixed greens
- 1/4 cup goat cheese, crumbled
- 1/4 cup walnuts, toasted
- 2 tablespoons balsamic vinaigrette
- Salt and pepper to taste

Instructions:

1. Preheat the oven to 400°F (200°C). Wrap beets in foil and roast for 30-40 minutes until tender. Let cool, then peel and slice.
2. In a large bowl, combine mixed greens, roasted beets, goat cheese, and walnuts.
3. Drizzle with balsamic vinaigrette, toss gently, and season with salt and pepper before serving.

Nutritional Information:

- Calories: 250; Fat: 15g; Protein: 7g; Carbs: 25g

Chia Seed Pudding with Berries

Benefits: Chia Seed Pudding with Berries is a nutrient-dense breakfast or snack. Chia seeds are high in omega-3 fatty acids and fiber, while berries add antioxidants and natural sweetness.

Servings: 4
Preparation Time: 5 minutes
Cooking Time: 0 minutes (overnight chilling)

Ingredients:

- 1/2 cup chia seeds
- 2 cups unsweetened almond milk
- 1 tablespoon maple syrup (optional)
- 1 teaspoon vanilla extract
- 1 cup mixed berries (strawberries, blueberries, raspberries)

Instructions:

1. In a bowl, mix chia seeds, almond milk, maple syrup, and vanilla extract. Stir well to avoid clumping.
2. Cover and refrigerate overnight or for at least 4 hours until thickened.
3. Serve topped with fresh berries.

Nutritional Information:

- Calories: 200; Fat: 10g; Protein: 6g; Carbs: 20g

Eggplant Parmesan

Benefits: Eggplant Parmesan is a comforting and hearty dish that provides a satisfying texture and flavor. Eggplant is low in calories and high in fiber, making it a great choice for weight management.

Servings: 4
Preparation Time: 20 minutes
Cooking Time: 40 minutes

Ingredients:

- 2 medium eggplants, sliced into rounds
- 1 cup whole wheat breadcrumbs
- 1 cup marinara sauce
- 1 cup mozzarella cheese, shredded
- 1/4 cup parmesan cheese, grated
- 1 teaspoon Italian seasoning
- 2 tablespoons olive oil
- Salt and pepper to taste

Instructions:

1. Preheat the oven to 375°F (190°C).
2. Sprinkle eggplant slices with salt and let sit for 10 minutes to draw out moisture. Rinse and pat dry.
3. In a bowl, combine breadcrumbs, Italian seasoning, salt, and pepper. Dip eggplant slices in olive oil, then coat with breadcrumb mixture.
4. Place on a baking sheet and bake for 20 minutes, flipping halfway through, until golden.
5. In a baking dish, layer marinara sauce, baked eggplant, mozzarella, and parmesan. Repeat layers, finishing with cheese on top.
6. Bake for an additional 20 minutes until cheese is bubbly and golden.

Nutritional Information:

- Calories: 350; Fat: 20g; Protein: 15g; Carbs: 30g

Apple Cinnamon Oatmeal

Benefits: Apple Cinnamon Oatmeal is a wholesome breakfast option that's filling and nutritious. Oats provide soluble fiber for heart health, while apples add natural sweetness and fiber.

Servings: 4
Preparation Time: 10 minutes
Cooking Time: 15 minutes

Ingredients:

- 2 cups rolled oats
- 4 cups water or unsweetened almond milk
- 2 apples, diced
- 1 teaspoon cinnamon
- 1 tablespoon maple syrup (optional)
- 1/4 cup walnuts, chopped (optional)

Instructions:

1. In a saucepan, bring water or almond milk to a boil.
2. Stir in oats, diced apples, and cinnamon. Reduce heat and simmer for about 10-15 minutes until oats are tender.
3. Sweeten with maple syrup if desired and serve topped with walnuts.

Nutritional Information:

- Calories: 300; Fat: 10g; Protein: 8g; Carbs: 50g

Avocado and Tomato Toast

Benefits: Avocado and Tomato Toast is a quick and nutritious meal that provides healthy fats and fiber. Avocados are rich in heart-healthy monounsaturated fats, while tomatoes offer antioxidants.

Servings: 2
Preparation Time: 5 minutes
Cooking Time: 0 minutes

Ingredients:

- 2 slices whole grain bread
- 1 ripe avocado
- 1 cup cherry tomatoes, halved
- 1 tablespoon lemon juice
- Salt and pepper to taste
- Fresh basil for garnish

Instructions:

1. Toast the whole grain bread until golden brown.
2. In a bowl, mash the avocado and mix in lemon juice, salt, and pepper.
3. Spread the avocado mixture onto the toasted bread.
4. Top with cherry tomatoes and garnish with fresh basil before serving.

Nutritional Information:

- Calories: 300; Fat: 15g; Protein: 6g; Carbs: 35g

Chapter 13 Whole Grains Recipes

Chapter 13 Whole Grains Recipes

Quinoa Salad with Lemon Vinaigrette

Benefits: This Quinoa Salad is packed with fresh vegetables and protein-rich quinoa, making it a perfect light meal. Quinoa is a complete protein, offering all nine essential amino acids, and its fiber content promotes digestive health.

Servings: 4
Preparation Time: 15 minutes
Cooking Time: 15 minutes

Ingredients:

- 1 cup quinoa
- 2 cups water
- 1 cucumber, diced
- 1 bell pepper, diced
- 1 cup cherry tomatoes, halved
- 1/4 cup red onion, finely chopped
- 1/4 cup fresh parsley, chopped
- 3 tablespoons olive oil
- Juice of 1 lemon
- Salt and pepper to taste

Instructions:

1. Rinse quinoa under cold water to remove bitterness.
2. In a saucepan, combine quinoa and water. Bring to a boil, then reduce to a simmer, cover, and cook for 15 minutes or until water is absorbed.
3. Fluff quinoa with a fork and let cool.
4. In a large bowl, combine cucumber, bell pepper, cherry tomatoes, red onion, and parsley.
5. In a small bowl, whisk together olive oil, lemon juice, salt, and pepper.
6. Add cooled quinoa to the vegetable mixture and pour dressing over. Toss well to combine.

Nutritional Information:

- Calories: 250; Fat: 10g; Protein: 8g; Carbs: 36g

Brown Rice Stir-Fry with Vegetables

Benefits: This Brown Rice Stir-Fry is a nutrient-dense dish that incorporates a variety of colorful vegetables. Brown rice is high in fiber and aids in maintaining healthy blood sugar levels, while the vegetables provide essential vitamins and minerals.

Servings: 4
Preparation Time: 10 minutes
Cooking Time: 20 minutes

Ingredients:

- 1 cup brown rice
- 2 cups water
- 1 tablespoon sesame oil
- 1 cup broccoli florets
- 1 cup bell pepper, sliced
- 1 cup carrots, julienned
- 2 cloves garlic, minced
- 1 tablespoon low-sodium soy sauce
- 1 tablespoon ginger, minced
- Green onions for garnish

Instructions:

1. Rinse brown rice under cold water. In a saucepan, combine rice and water. Bring to a boil, reduce heat, cover, and simmer for about 45 minutes or until rice is tender.
2. Heat sesame oil in a large skillet over medium heat. Add garlic and ginger, sauté for 1 minute.
3. Add broccoli, bell pepper, and carrots. Stir-fry for 5-7 minutes until tender-crisp.
4. Stir in cooked brown rice and soy sauce. Mix well and cook for another 2 minutes.
5. Garnish with sliced green onions before serving.

Nutritional Information:

- Calories: 300; Fat: 10g; Protein: 8g; Carbs: 52g

Whole Wheat Pasta with Spinach and Garlic

Benefits: Whole Wheat Pasta with Spinach and Garlic is a simple yet satisfying meal. Whole wheat pasta provides complex carbohydrates for sustained energy, while spinach is rich in iron and antioxidants, supporting overall health.

Servings: 4
Preparation Time: 10 minutes
Cooking Time: 15 minutes

Ingredients:

- 12 oz whole wheat pasta
- 3 tablespoons olive oil
- 4 cloves garlic, minced
- 5 cups fresh spinach
- 1/4 teaspoon red pepper flakes (optional)
- Salt and pepper to taste
- 1/4 cup grated Parmesan cheese (optional)

Instructions:

1. Cook whole wheat pasta according to package instructions. Drain and set aside.
2. In a large skillet, heat olive oil over medium heat. Add minced garlic and red pepper flakes; sauté for 1 minute.
3. Add fresh spinach to the skillet and cook until wilted, about 3-4 minutes.
4. Toss in the cooked pasta, mixing well to combine. Season with salt and pepper.
5. Serve warm, topped with grated Parmesan cheese if desired.

Nutritional Information:

- Calories: 350; Fat: 15g; Protein: 12g; Carbs: 50g

Barley and Mushroom Risotto

Benefits: Barley and Mushroom Risotto is a creamy, comforting dish that's naturally gluten-free. Barley is high in fiber and beneficial for heart health, while mushrooms add umami flavor and essential nutrients.

Servings: 4
Preparation Time: 10 minutes
Cooking Time: 30 minutes

Ingredients:

- 1 cup pearl barley
- 4 cups vegetable broth
- 1 cup mushrooms, sliced
- 1 onion, diced
- 2 cloves garlic, minced
- 1/2 cup peas (fresh or frozen)
- 2 tablespoons olive oil
- 1/4 teaspoon thyme
- Salt and pepper to taste

Instructions:

1. In a pot, heat vegetable broth and keep it warm.
2. In a separate pan, heat olive oil over medium heat. Add onion and garlic, sauté until translucent.
3. Stir in mushrooms and cook for 5 minutes until softened.
4. Add barley, stirring to coat. Pour in 1 cup of warm broth and stir until absorbed.
5. Continue adding broth, one cup at a time, stirring frequently until barley is tender (about 25-30 minutes).
6. Stir in peas and thyme during the last few minutes of cooking. Season with salt and pepper before serving.

Nutritional Information:

- Calories: 320; Fat: 8g; Protein: 12g; Carbs: 55g

Oatmeal with Bananas and Almonds

Benefits: Oatmeal with Bananas and Almonds is a hearty breakfast option rich in fiber. Oats are known for their heart-healthy benefits, while bananas provide potassium and natural sweetness.

Servings: 4
Preparation Time: 5 minutes
Cooking Time: 10 minutes

Ingredients:

- 2 cups rolled oats
- 4 cups water or unsweetened almond milk
- 2 ripe bananas, sliced
- 1/4 cup almonds, chopped
- 1 teaspoon cinnamon
- 1 tablespoon maple syrup (optional)

Instructions:

1. In a saucepan, bring water or almond milk to a boil.
2. Stir in rolled oats and reduce heat. Cook for 5-7 minutes until creamy, stirring occasionally.
3. Mix in sliced bananas, cinnamon, and maple syrup if desired.
4. Serve topped with chopped almonds for crunch.

Nutritional Information:

- Calories: 350; Fat: 12g; Protein: 10g; Carbs: 55g

Millet and Vegetable Pilaf

Benefits: Millet and Vegetable Pilaf is a versatile dish that's naturally gluten-free. Millet is a nutritious grain high in magnesium, and the variety of vegetables adds essential vitamins and minerals.

Servings: 4
Preparation Time: 10 minutes
Cooking Time: 20 minutes

Ingredients:

- 1 cup millet
- 2 cups vegetable broth
- 1 carrot, diced
- 1 zucchini, diced
- 1 red bell pepper, diced
- 1 onion, diced
- 2 tablespoons olive oil
- Salt and pepper to taste
- Fresh parsley for garnish

Instructions:

1. Rinse millet under cold water.
2. In a saucepan, heat olive oil over medium heat. Add onion and sauté until translucent.
3. Stir in carrots, zucchini, and bell pepper. Cook for 5-7 minutes.
4. Add millet and vegetable broth. Bring to a boil, reduce heat, cover, and simmer for about 15 minutes or until millet is tender and broth is absorbed.
5. Fluff with a fork, season with salt and pepper, and garnish with parsley before serving.

Nutritional Information:

- Calories: 290; Fat: 8g; Protein: 9g; Carbs: 50g

Whole Wheat Berry Salad with Feta

Benefits: Whole Wheat Berry Salad with Feta is a refreshing dish rich in fiber and protein. Wheat berries are a whole grain powerhouse, and this salad is perfect as a side or main dish.

Servings: 4
Preparation Time: 15 minutes
Cooking Time: 25 minutes

Ingredients:

- 1 cup wheat berries
- 4 cups water
- 1 cup cherry tomatoes, halved
- 1 cucumber, diced
- 1/2 cup feta cheese, crumbled
- 1/4 cup fresh basil, chopped
- 2 tablespoons olive oil
- Juice of 1 lemon
- Salt and pepper to taste

Instructions:

1. Rinse wheat berries under cold water. In a pot, combine wheat berries and water. Bring to a boil, then reduce heat and simmer for about 25 minutes until tender.
2. Drain excess water and let cool.
3. In a large bowl, combine cooked wheat berries, cherry tomatoes, cucumber, feta, and basil.
4. In a small bowl, whisk together olive oil, lemon juice, salt, and pepper.
5. Pour dressing over salad and toss to combine.

Nutritional Information:

- Calories: 350; Fat: 14g; Protein: 12g; Carbs: 48g

Spelt Pancakes with Berries

Benefits: Spelt Pancakes with Berries are a delicious breakfast option packed with antioxidants. Spelt is an ancient grain rich in protein and fiber, making these pancakes a nutritious start to the day.

Servings: 4
Preparation Time: 10 minutes
Cooking Time: 15 minutes

Ingredients:

- 1 cup spelt flour
- 1 tablespoon baking powder
- 1 tablespoon cinnamon
- 1 cup almond milk
- 1 tablespoon maple syrup (optional)
- 1 cup mixed berries (fresh or frozen)

Instructions:

1. In a bowl, combine spelt flour, baking powder, and cinnamon.
2. In another bowl, whisk together almond milk and maple syrup.
3. Combine wet and dry ingredients, mixing until just combined. Gently fold in berries.
4. Heat a non-stick skillet over medium heat and pour 1/4 cup batter for each pancake. Cook until bubbles form, then flip and cook until golden.
5. Serve warm with additional berries on top.

Nutritional Information:

- Calories: 250; Fat: 6g; Protein: 8g; Carbs: 44g

Farro Bowl with Roasted Vegetables

Benefits: Farro Bowl with Roasted Vegetables is a hearty, nutrient-rich dish. Farro is a great source of fiber and protein, and roasting vegetables enhances their natural sweetness and flavor.

Servings: 4
Preparation Time: 15 minutes
Cooking Time: 25 minutes

Ingredients:

- 4 cups water
- 1 zucchini, diced
- 1 red bell pepper, diced
- 1 cup Brussels sprouts, halved
- 2 tablespoons olive oil
- Salt and pepper to taste
- 1/4 teaspoon garlic pow
- 1 cup farroder

Instructions:

1. Rinse farro under cold water. In a pot, combine farro and water. Bring to a boil, reduce heat, and simmer for about 25-30 minutes until tender.
2. Preheat oven to 400°F (200°C). On a baking sheet, toss zucchini, bell pepper, and Brussels sprouts with olive oil, garlic powder, salt, and pepper. Roast for 20 minutes until tender.
3. To serve, place cooked farro in bowls and top with roasted vegetables.

Nutritional Information:

- Calories: 360; Fat: 12g; Protein: 14g; Carbs: 54g

Chia Seed Pudding with Almond Milk

Benefits: Chia Seed Pudding with Almond Milk is a satisfying and nutritious breakfast or snack. Chia seeds are packed with omega-3 fatty acids, fiber, and protein, providing lasting energy and fullness.

Servings: 4
Preparation Time: 10 minutes
Cooking Time: 0 minutes (refrigerate overnight)

Ingredients:

- 1/2 cup chia seeds
- 2 cups unsweetened almond milk
- 1 teaspoon vanilla extract
- 1 tablespoon maple syrup (optional)
- Fresh fruits for topping (berries, banana, etc.)

Instructions:

1. In a bowl, combine chia seeds, almond milk, vanilla extract, and maple syrup. Stir well to prevent clumping.
2. Cover and refrigerate for at least 4 hours or overnight until thickened.
3. Before serving, stir the pudding and top with fresh fruits.

Nutritional Information:

- Calories: 180; Fat: 9g; Protein: 6g; Carbs: 24g

Buckwheat and Vegetable Soup

Benefits: Buckwheat and Vegetable Soup is a comforting and nourishing option. Buckwheat is gluten-free and rich in antioxidants, making this soup a perfect choice for maintaining overall health.

Servings: 4
Preparation Time: 15 minutes
Cooking Time: 30 minutes

Ingredients:

- 1 cup buckwheat
- 4 cups vegetable broth
- 1 carrot, diced
- 1 celery stalk, diced
- 1 onion, diced
- 2 cloves garlic, minced
- 1 cup kale, chopped
- 1 tablespoon olive oil
- Salt and pepper to taste

Instructions:

1. Rinse buckwheat under cold water.
2. In a large pot, heat olive oil over medium heat. Add onion, carrot, celery, and garlic; sauté until softened.
3. Pour in vegetable broth and add buckwheat. Bring to a boil, reduce heat, and simmer for 15-20 minutes.
4. Stir in chopped kale and cook until wilted. Season with salt and pepper before serving.

Nutritional Information:

- Calories: 220; Fat: 6g; Protein: 10g; Carbs: 36g

Whole Grain Tortilla Wraps with Hummus

Benefits: Whole Grain Tortilla Wraps with Hummus are a quick and nutritious meal. Whole grain tortillas provide fiber, while hummus adds protein and healthy fats, making this wrap satisfying and delicious.

Servings: 4
Preparation Time: 10 minutes
Cooking Time: 0 minutes

Ingredients:

- 4 whole grain tortillas
- 1 cup hummus
- 1 cup spinach leaves
- 1 bell pepper, sliced
- 1 cucumber, sliced
- 1 carrot, grated

Instructions:

1. Spread 1/4 cup hummus on each tortilla.
2. Layer spinach, bell pepper, cucumber, and grated carrot on top.
3. Roll the tortilla tightly and slice in half before serving.

Nutritional Information:

- Calories: 280; Fat: 8g; Protein: 10g; Carbs: 44g

Teff Porridge with Apple and Cinnamon

Benefits: Teff Porridge with Apple and Cinnamon is a warm, hearty breakfast. Teff is a nutrient-rich grain high in protein and calcium, while apples provide natural sweetness and fiber.

Servings: 4
Preparation Time: 5 minutes
Cooking Time: 15 minutes

Ingredients:

- 1 cup teff
- 4 cups water
- 2 apples, diced
- 1 teaspoon cinnamon
- 1 tablespoon maple syrup (optional)
- Chopped nuts for topping

Instructions:

1. Rinse teff under cold water. In a saucepan, combine teff and water. Bring to a boil, then reduce heat and simmer for about 15 minutes until cooked.
2. Stir in diced apples, cinnamon, and maple syrup (if using). Cook for another 5 minutes.
3. Serve warm, topped with chopped nuts.

Nutritional Information:

- Calories: 290; Fat: 6g; Protein: 10g; Carbs: 52g

Freekeh Salad with Roasted Chickpeas

Benefits: Freekeh Salad with Roasted Chickpeas is a protein-packed dish with a variety of textures. Freekeh is high in fiber and nutrients, making this salad both filling and satisfying.

Servings: 4
Preparation Time: 15 minutes
Cooking Time: 30 minutes

Ingredients:

- 1 cup freekeh
- 4 cups water
- 1 can chickpeas, drained and rinsed
- 2 tablespoons olive oil
- 1 teaspoon paprika
- 1 teaspoon cumin
- 1 cucumber, diced
- 1 cup cherry tomatoes, halved
- Salt and pepper to taste

Instructions:

1. Rinse freekeh under cold water. In a pot, combine freekeh and water. Bring to a boil, then reduce heat and simmer for about 25 minutes until tender.
2. Preheat oven to 400°F (200°C). On a baking sheet, toss chickpeas with olive oil, paprika, cumin, salt, and pepper. Roast for 20-25 minutes until crispy.
3. In a large bowl, combine cooked freekeh, cucumber, cherry tomatoes, and roasted chickpeas. Mix well and adjust seasoning if necessary.

Nutritional Information:

- Calories: 400; Fat: 14g; Protein: 15g; Carbs: 58g

Quinoa Breakfast Bowl with Nuts and Seeds

Benefits: Quinoa Breakfast Bowl with Nuts and Seeds is a nourishing start to your day. Quinoa provides protein and fiber, while the combination of nuts and seeds adds healthy fats and crunch.

Servings: 4
Preparation Time: 10 minutes
Cooking Time: 15 minutes

Ingredients:

- 1 cup quinoa
- 2 cups almond milk
- 1/4 cup walnuts, chopped
- 1/4 cup pumpkin seeds
- 2 tablespoons chia seeds
- 1 tablespoon maple syrup (optional)
- Fresh fruit for topping

Instructions:

1. Rinse quinoa under cold water. In a saucepan, combine quinoa and almond milk. Bring to a boil, then reduce heat and simmer for about 15 minutes until liquid is absorbed.
2. Stir in walnuts, pumpkin seeds, chia seeds, and maple syrup (if using).
3. Serve warm, topped with fresh fruit.

Nutritional Information:

- Calories: 360; Fat: 18g; Protein: 12g; Carbs: 42g

Chapter 14 Fruits Recipes

Chapter 14 Fruits Recipes

Tropical Fruit Salad with Lime Dressing

Benefits: Tropical Fruit Salad with Lime Dressing is a refreshing and hydrating dish, perfect for warm days. Packed with vitamins, antioxidants, and hydration, this salad supports immune function and overall health.

Servings: 4
Preparation Time: 15 minutes
Cooking Time: 0 minutes

Ingredients:

- 1 cup pineapple, diced
- 1 cup mango, diced
- 1 cup kiwi, peeled and sliced
- 1 cup strawberries, halved
- 1 cup blueberries
- 2 tablespoons fresh lime juice
- 1 tablespoon honey (optional)
- Fresh mint leaves for garnish

Instructions:

1. In a large bowl, combine pineapple, mango, kiwi, strawberries, and blueberries.
2. In a small bowl, whisk together lime juice and honey (if using).
3. Drizzle the lime dressing over the fruit and gently toss to combine.
4. Serve chilled, garnished with fresh mint leaves.

Nutritional Information:

- Calories: 150; Fat: 0.5g; Protein: 2g; Carbs: 38g

Avocado and Mango Salsa

Benefits: Avocado and Mango Salsa is not only delicious but also rich in healthy fats and vitamins. The combination of avocado and mango provides a burst of flavor and nutrients, making it a perfect addition to any meal.

Servings: 4
Preparation Time: 10 minutes
Cooking Time: 0 minutes

Ingredients:

- 1 ripe avocado, diced
- 1 cup mango, diced
- 1/2 red onion, finely chopped
- 1 jalapeño, seeded and minced
- 1/4 cup fresh cilantro, chopped
- 1 lime, juiced
- Salt to taste

Instructions:

1. In a medium bowl, combine avocado, mango, red onion, jalapeño, and cilantro.
2. Drizzle lime juice over the mixture and gently toss.
3. Season with salt to taste. Serve immediately with whole grain tortilla chips or as a topping for grilled chicken.

Nutritional Information:

- Calories: 180; Fat: 10g; Protein: 3g; Carbs: 25g

Berry Chia Pudding

Benefits: Berry Chia Pudding is a nutritious and filling breakfast or snack option. Packed with fiber, omega-3 fatty acids, and antioxidants, this pudding supports digestion and heart health.

Servings: 4
Preparation Time: 10 minutes
Cooking Time: 0 minutes (requires refrigeration)

Ingredients:

- 1/2 cup chia seeds
- 2 cups almond milk (unsweetened)
- 1 cup mixed berries (strawberries, blueberries, raspberries)
- 1 tablespoon vanilla extract
- 1 tablespoon maple syrup (optional)

Instructions:

1. In a bowl, whisk together chia seeds, almond milk, vanilla extract, and maple syrup (if using).
2. Cover and refrigerate for at least 4 hours or overnight until it thickens.
3. Before serving, stir well and layer with mixed berries in serving glasses.

Nutritional Information:

- Calories: 200; Fat: 9g; Protein: 6g; Carbs: 28g

Watermelon and Feta Salad

Benefits: Watermelon and Feta Salad is a refreshing and hydrating dish, perfect for summer. Watermelon is rich in vitamins A and C, while feta adds a savory touch and protein.

Servings: 4
Preparation Time: 10 minutes
Cooking Time: 0 minutes

Ingredients:

- 4 cups watermelon, cubed
- 1 cup feta cheese, crumbled
- 1/4 red onion, thinly sliced
- 1/4 cup fresh mint leaves, chopped
- 2 tablespoons balsamic vinegar
- Salt and pepper to taste

Instructions:

1. In a large bowl, combine watermelon, feta cheese, red onion, and mint leaves.
2. Drizzle balsamic vinegar over the salad and season with salt and pepper.
3. Gently toss to combine and serve chilled.

Nutritional Information:

- Calories: 170; Fat: 8g; Protein: 5g; Carbs: 20g

Baked Apple with Cinnamon and Nuts

Benefits: Baked Apple with Cinnamon and Nuts is a warm and comforting dessert rich in fiber and healthy fats. This dish is perfect for satisfying your sweet tooth without added sugars.

Servings: 4
Preparation Time: 10 minutes
Cooking Time: 20 minutes

Ingredients:

- 4 medium apples, cored
- 1/2 cup walnuts, chopped
- 1 teaspoon cinnamon
- 2 tablespoons maple syrup (optional)
- 1/4 cup raisins (optional)

Instructions:

1. Preheat the oven to 350°F (175°C).
2. Place cored apples in a baking dish.
3. In a bowl, mix walnuts, cinnamon, maple syrup (if using), and raisins (if using).
4. Stuff the mixture into the center of each apple.
5. Bake for 20 minutes until apples are tender. Serve warm.

Nutritional Information:

- Calories: 220; Fat: 10g; Protein: 3g; Carbs: 36g

Citrus Quinoa Salad

Benefits: Citrus Quinoa Salad is a vibrant dish packed with vitamin C and protein. Quinoa is a complete protein, making this salad a nutritious choice for a light lunch or dinner.

Servings: 4
Preparation Time: 15 minutes
Cooking Time: 15 minutes

Ingredients:

- 1 cup quinoa
- 2 cups water
- 1 orange, segmented
- 1 grapefruit, segmented
- 1/4 cup almonds, sliced
- 1 tablespoon olive oil
- Salt and pepper to taste

Instructions:

1. Rinse quinoa under cold water. In a pot, combine quinoa and water. Bring to a boil, reduce heat, and simmer for about 15 minutes until liquid is absorbed.
2. In a large bowl, combine cooked quinoa, orange segments, grapefruit segments, and sliced almonds.
3. Drizzle olive oil and season with salt and pepper. Gently toss to combine. Serve warm or chilled.

Nutritional Information:

- Calories: 280; Fat: 10g; Protein: 8g; Carbs: 44g

Frozen Banana Bites

Benefits: Frozen Banana Bites are a delightful and healthy treat. They combine the energy-boosting properties of bananas with antioxidant-rich dark chocolate, making for a satisfying snack.

Servings: 4
Preparation Time: 10 minutes
Cooking Time: 0 minutes (requires freezing)

Ingredients:

- 2 ripe bananas, sliced
- 1/2 cup dark chocolate (70% cocoa or higher), melted
- 1/4 cup crushed nuts (almonds, walnuts, or pistachios)

Instructions:

1. Line a baking sheet with parchment paper.
2. Dip banana slices into melted dark chocolate, coating them evenly.
3. Place the coated banana slices on the prepared baking sheet and sprinkle with crushed nuts.
4. Freeze for at least 2 hours until firm. Serve frozen.

Nutritional Information:

- Calories: 200; Fat: 12g; Protein: 3g; Carbs: 25g

Pear and Walnut Salad

Benefits: Pear and Walnut Salad is a nutrient-rich dish loaded with fiber and healthy fats. This salad provides a perfect balance of sweetness and crunch, ideal for lunch or dinner.

Servings: 4
Preparation Time: 10 minutes
Cooking Time: 0 minutes

Ingredients:

- 4 cups mixed greens (spinach, arugula, etc.)
- 2 ripe pears, sliced
- 1/2 cup walnuts, toasted
- 1/4 cup goat cheese, crumbled
- 2 tablespoons balsamic vinaigrette

Instructions:

1. In a large bowl, combine mixed greens, sliced pears, toasted walnuts, and goat cheese.
2. Drizzle with balsamic vinaigrette and gently toss to combine.
3. Serve immediately.

Nutritional Information:

- Calories: 280; Fat: 18g; Protein: 6g; Carbs: 30g

Smoothie Bowl with Spinach and Bananas

Benefits: Smoothie Bowl with Spinach and Bananas is a delicious and nutritious breakfast option. This recipe is rich in vitamins, minerals, and fiber, making it an excellent way to start your day.

Servings: 2
Preparation Time: 10 minutes
Cooking Time: 0 minutes

Ingredients:

- 2 ripe bananas
- 1 cup spinach
- 1 cup almond milk (unsweetened)
- 1 tablespoon peanut butter (optional)
- Toppings: sliced fruits, chia seeds, granola

Instructions:

1. In a blender, combine bananas, spinach, almond milk, and peanut butter (if using). Blend until smooth.
2. Pour the smoothie into bowls and top with sliced fruits, chia seeds, and granola. Serve immediately.

Nutritional Information:

- Calories: 350; Fat: 12g; Protein: 10g; Carbs: 50g

Grilled Peaches with Honey

Benefits: Grilled Peaches with Honey is a simple yet indulgent dessert. Peaches are high in vitamins A and C, while grilling enhances their natural sweetness without added sugars.

Servings: 4
Preparation Time: 5 minutes
Cooking Time: 5 minutes

Ingredients:

- 4 ripe peaches, halved and pitted
- 2 tablespoons olive oil
- 2 tablespoons honey (optional)
- 1/4 cup Greek yogurt (optional)

Instructions:

1. Preheat a grill or grill pan over medium heat.
2. Brush peach halves with olive oil and place them cut side down on the grill.
3. Grill for about 4-5 minutes until grill marks appear and peaches are softened.
4. Drizzle with honey and serve warm, optionally topped with Greek yogurt.

Nutritional Information:

- Calories: 180; Fat: 7g; Protein: 3g; Carbs: 30g

Coconut and Pineapple Energy Bites

Benefits: Coconut and Pineapple Energy Bites are a perfect on-the-go snack. These bites provide a quick energy boost with healthy fats, fiber, and natural sweetness, making them ideal for workouts or busy days.

Servings: 12
Preparation Time: 15 minutes
Cooking Time: 0 minutes

Ingredients:

- 1 cup dates, pitted
- 1/2 cup almonds
- 1/2 cup unsweetened shredded coconut
- 1/2 cup dried pineapple, chopped
- 1 tablespoon chia seeds

Instructions:

1. In a food processor, combine dates, almonds, shredded coconut, dried pineapple, and chia seeds. Blend until the mixture is sticky and holds together.
2. Roll the mixture into bite-sized balls and place them on a baking sheet.
3. Refrigerate for at least 30 minutes to firm up before serving.

Nutritional Information:

- Calories: 100; Fat: 5g; Protein: 2g; Carbs: 12g

Chocolate Avocado Mousse

Benefits: Chocolate Avocado Mousse is a rich and decadent dessert that's actually good for you. Avocados provide healthy fats and fiber, while cocoa powder is packed with antioxidants.

Servings: 4
Preparation Time: 10 minutes
Cooking Time: 0 minutes (requires chilling)

Ingredients:

- 2 ripe avocados
- 1/2 cup unsweetened cocoa powder
- 1/4 cup maple syrup (adjust to taste)
- 1/4 cup almond milk (unsweetened)
- 1 teaspoon vanilla extract

Instructions:

1. In a blender, combine avocados, cocoa powder, maple syrup, almond milk, and vanilla extract. Blend until smooth and creamy.
2. Adjust sweetness to taste by adding more maple syrup if desired.
3. Spoon the mousse into serving bowls and refrigerate for at least 30 minutes before serving.

Nutritional Information:

- Calories: 220; Fat: 14g; Protein: 3g; Carbs: 28g

Strawberry Banana Overnight Oats

Benefits: Strawberry Banana Overnight Oats are a convenient and nutritious breakfast. Packed with fiber and protein, this dish keeps you full and energized throughout the morning.

Servings: 2
Preparation Time: 10 minutes (requires overnight chilling)
Cooking Time: 0 minutes

Ingredients:

- 1 cup rolled oats
- 2 cups almond milk (unsweetened)
- 1 ripe banana, sliced
- 1 cup strawberries, sliced
- 1 tablespoon chia seeds
- 1 tablespoon almond butter (optional)

Instructions:

1. In a bowl, combine rolled oats, almond milk, chia seeds, and almond butter (if using). Stir well.
2. Divide the mixture into two jars and layer with sliced bananas and strawberries.
3. Cover and refrigerate overnight. Serve cold in the morning.

Nutritional Information:

- Calories: 350; Fat: 10g; Protein: 12g; Carbs: 55g

Raspberry Almond Smoothie

Benefits: Raspberry Almond Smoothie is a delicious and refreshing way to enjoy your fruits. Rich in antioxidants, healthy fats, and fiber, this smoothie supports heart health and digestion.

Servings: 2
Preparation Time: 5 minutes
Cooking Time: 0 minutes

Ingredients:

- 1 cup fresh raspberries
- 1 ripe banana
- 1/2 cup almond milk (unsweetened)
- 1 tablespoon almond butter
- 1 tablespoon flaxseeds (optional)

Instructions:

1. In a blender, combine raspberries, banana, almond milk, almond butter, and flaxseeds (if using).
2. Blend until smooth and creamy. Adjust sweetness if necessary.
3. Pour into glasses and serve immediately.

Nutritional Information:

- Calories: 220; Fat: 10g; Protein: 6g; Carbs: 30g

Papaya Salad with Lime and Mint

Benefits: Papaya Salad with Lime and Mint is a light and refreshing dish full of vitamins and antioxidants. Papaya aids digestion and provides a tropical flair to your meals.

Servings: 4
Preparation Time: 10 minutes
Cooking Time: 0 minutes

Ingredients:

- 2 cups ripe papaya, diced
- 1/4 cup red onion, thinly sliced
- 1/4 cup fresh mint leaves, chopped
- 1 lime, juiced
- Salt to taste

Instructions:

1. In a large bowl, combine diced papaya, red onion, and mint leaves.
2. Drizzle lime juice over the salad and season with salt.
3. Gently toss to combine and serve chilled.

Nutritional Information:

- Calories: 90; Fat: 0g; Protein: 1g; Carbs: 23g

Chapter 14 Recipes Index

Chapter 15 Conclusion

In conclusion, Good Energy nutrition represents a transformative approach to eating that prioritizes whole, nutrient-dense foods for optimal health and well-being. Rooted in the teachings of Dr. Casey Means, this dietary framework emphasizes the importance of understanding how different foods impact energy levels, metabolism, and overall health. By adopting the principles of Good Energy nutrition, individuals can experience numerous benefits, including sustained energy, improved metabolic health, effective weight management, enhanced mental clarity, and holistic well-being.

The key to successfully implementing the Good Energy diet lies in focusing on whole foods, balancing macronutrients, staying hydrated, and practicing mindful eating. These principles not only enhance the physical aspects of health but also contribute to a more satisfying and enjoyable eating experience.

As individuals embark on their journey with Good Energy nutrition, it is essential to recognize that this approach is not about perfection but rather about progress. Small, sustainable changes can lead to significant improvements in health and well-being over time. By committing to this dietary framework, you can unlock your full potential and experience the vibrant energy and vitality that comes from nourishing your body with intention and care.

Ultimately, Good Energy nutrition is about more than just food; it's about cultivating a lifestyle that values health, happiness, and vitality. It empowers individuals to take control of their dietary choices and fosters a greater connection to the nourishment that food provides. With dedication and mindfulness, the principles of Good Energy nutrition can serve as a powerful ally in achieving lasting health and wellness.

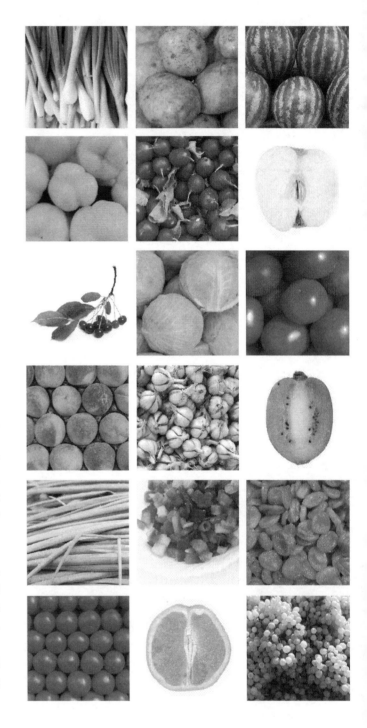

Made in the USA
Monee, IL
23 December 2024

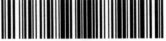

75220827R00050